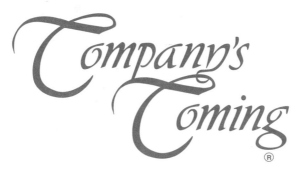

Easy Healthy Recipes

Jean Paré

www.companyscoming.com
visit our ↰website

Front Cover

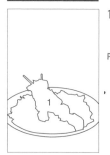

1. Minted Beef and
   Noodles, page 46

Props courtesy of: Chintz &
Company

Back Cover

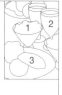

1. Poppy Seed Fruit Bowl,
   page 23
2. Creamy Raspberry Cool
   page 12
3. Fruit-Full Muffins,
   page 148

Props courtesy of: Casa Bugatti
Stokes

Sixth Printing May 2011

Library and Archives Canada Cataloguing in Publication

Paré, Jean, date-
Easy healthy recipes /Jean Paré.
(Original series)
Includes index.
ISBN 978-1-897477-28-1
1. Cookery. 2. Cookery (Fruit).
3. Cookery (Vegetables).
I. Title. II. Series: Paré, Jean, date- . Original series.
TX715.6.P3555 2009   641.5   C2009-901447-5

We gratefully acknowledge the following suppliers for their generous support of our Test and Photography Kitchens:

Broil King Barbecues
Hamilton Beach® Canada
Proctor Silex® Canada
Corelle®
Lagostina®
Tupperware®

Published by
Company's Coming Publishing Limited
2311 – 96 Street
Edmonton, Alberta, Canada T6N 1G3
Tel: 780-450-6223   Fax: 780-450-1857
www.companyscoming.com

Company's Coming is a registered trademark owned by Company's Coming Publishing Limited

We acknowledge the financial support of the Government of Canada through the Canada Book Fund for our publishing activities.

Printed in China

Get more great recipes...FREE!

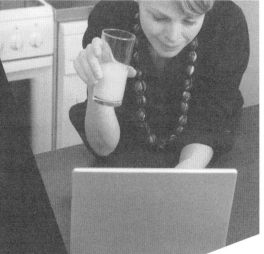

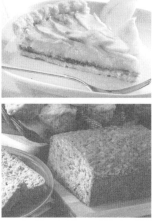

click

search

print

cook

From apple pie to zucchini bread, we've got you covered. Browse our free online recipes for Guaranteed Great!™ results.

You can also sign up to receive our **FREE online newsletter**. You'll receive exclusive offers, FREE recipes & cooking tips, new title previews, and much more...all delivered to your in-box.

So don't delay, visit our website today!

www.companyscoming.com
visit our ➤ website

Company's Coming Cookbooks

Quick & easy recipes; everyday ingredients!

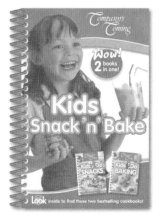

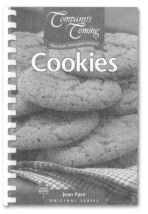

2-in-1 Cookbook Collection

- Softcover, 256 pages
- Lay-flat plastic coil binding
- Full-colour photos
- Nutrition information

Original Series

- Softcover, 160 pages
- Lay-flat plastic comb binding
- Full-colour photos
- Updated format

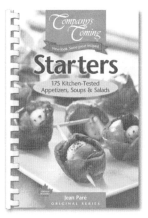

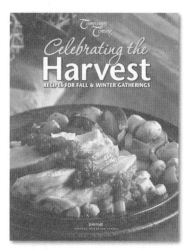

Original Series

- Softcover, 160 pages
- Lay-flat plastic comb binding
- Full-colour photos
- Nutrition information

Special Occasion Series

- Softcover, 176 pages
- Full-colour photos
- Nutrition information

For a complete listing of our cookbooks, visit our website:
www.companyscoming.com

Table of Contents

The Company's Coming Story

Jean Paré (pronounced "jeen PAIR-ee") grew up understanding that the combination of family, friends and home cooking is the best recipe for a good life. From her mother, she learned to appreciate good cooking, while her father praised even her earliest attempts in the kitchen. When Jean left home, she took with her a love of cooking, many family recipes and an intriguing desire to read cookbooks as if they were novels!

> *"Never share a recipe you wouldn't use yourself."*

When her four children had all reached school age, Jean volunteered to cater the 50th anniversary celebration of the Vermilion School of Agriculture, now Lakeland College, in Alberta, Canada. Working out of her home, Jean prepared a dinner for more than 1,000 people, launching a flourishing catering operation that continued for over 18 years. During that time, she had countless opportunities to test new ideas with immediate feedback—resulting in empty plates and contented customers! Whether preparing cocktail sandwiches for a house party or serving a hot meal for 1,500 people, Jean Paré earned a reputation for great food, courteous service and reasonable prices.

As requests for her recipes increased, Jean was often asked the question, "Why don't you write a cookbook?" Jean responded by teaming up with her son, Grant Lovig, in the fall of 1980 to form Company's Coming Publishing Limited. The publication of *150 Delicious Squares* on April 14, 1981 marked the debut of what would soon become one of the world's most popular cookbook series.

The company has grown since those early days when Jean worked from a spare bedroom in her home. Today, she continues to write recipes while working closely with the staff of the Recipe Factory, as the Company's Coming test kitchen is affectionately known.

There she fills the role of mentor, assisting with the development of recipes people most want to use for everyday cooking and easy entertaining. Every Company's Coming recipe is *kitchen-tested* before it is approved for publication.

Jean's daughter, Gail Lovig, is responsible for marketing and distribution, leading a team that includes sales personnel located in major cities across Canada. Company's Coming cookbooks are distributed in Canada, the United States, Australia and other world markets. Bestsellers many times over in English, Company's Coming cookbooks have also been published in French and Spanish.

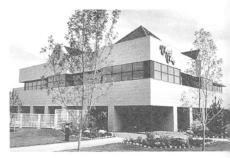

Familiar and trusted in home kitchens around the world, Company's Coming cookbooks are offered in a variety of formats. Highly regarded as kitchen workbooks, the softcover Original Series, with its lay-flat plastic comb binding, is still a favourite among readers.

Jean Paré's approach to cooking has always called for *quick and easy recipes* using *everyday ingredients*. That view has served her well. The recipient of many awards, including the Queen Elizabeth Golden Jubilee Medal, Jean was appointed Member of the Order of Canada, her country's highest lifetime achievement honour.

Jean continues to gain new supporters by adhering to what she calls The Golden Rule of Cooking: *Never share a recipe you wouldn't use yourself.* It's an approach that has worked—*millions of times over!*

Foreword

A healthy lifestyle doesn't mean we need to climb mountains, run marathons, or follow the latest fad diet. It means eating well and staying active if we want to feel better and have more energy.

It makes sense that a balanced diet is a good place to start. But what are the right foods to choose? *Canada's Food Guide to Healthy Eating* (page 9) outlines the average nutritional needs of a healthy diet. One particular recommendation caught our attention and became the focus of *Easy Healthy Recipes*.

Eating lots of fruit and vegetables is a key element to reducing health risks such as heart disease and cancer. When cooking for the family though, it can be a struggle to stay on track, particularly when it comes to meeting the recommended 5 to 10 servings of fruit and vegetables a day.

Easy Healthy Recipes offers a wide selection of dishes, each emphasizing fibre-rich fruit and vegetables. In fact, each recipe includes at least one full fruit or vegetable serving per portion. We've used this icon to identify those recipes with multiple fruit or vegetable servings.

The recipes themselves are lower in salt, fat and sugar, plus they're simple to prepare and adventurous in variety and taste. Some use more common vegetables like green beans, zucchini and squash, while others explore the intriguing tastes of less familiar vegetables like bok choy, eggplant and fennel. Or choose from an assortment of recipes using fruit—its sweet flavour offering just the right touch to beverages, soups, salads, main dishes, desserts and snacks.

Long-standing advice that we eat all our vegetables, or that an apple a day keeps the doctor away, may not be far wrong.

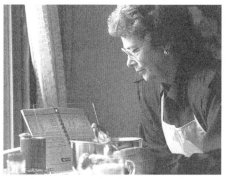

Healthy eating is the first step to living stronger and better. *Easy Healthy Recipes*— the title says it all. Every dish is a step in the right direction.

Jean Paré

Nutrition Information Guidelines

Each recipe is analyzed using the most current version of the Canadian Nutrient File from Health Canada, which is based on the United States Department of Agriculture (USDA) Nutrient Database.

- *If more than one ingredient is listed (such as "hard margarine or butter"), or if a range is (1 – 2 tsp., 5 – 10 mL), only the first ingredient or first amount is analyzed.*

- *For meat, poultry and fish, the serving size per person is based on the recommended 4 oz. (113 g) uncooked weight (without bone), which is 2 – 3 oz. (57 – 85 g) cooked weight (without bone)— approximately the size of a deck of playing cards.*

- *Milk used is 1% M.F. (milk fat), unless otherwise stated.*

- *Cooking oil used is canola oil, unless otherwise stated.*

- *Ingredients indicating "sprinkle," "optional," or "for garnish" are not included in the nutrition information.*

Margaret Ng, B.Sc. (Hon.), M.A.

Registered Dietitian

Common-Sense Eating

Healthy eating is all about making wise food choices, watching portion sizes and getting lots of variety.

Daily choices

Balance your meals and eat throughout the day. That means starting with breakfast—even something simple like a bowl of enriched cereal with fruit. Try to limit your caffeine intake each day. And don't forget, water is still your best thirst quencher. A mid-morning snack is a good idea, but reach for something healthy like a fruit or vegetable. Skipping lunch can often leave you with less energy in the afternoon. Plan to eat something nutritious at lunchtime to give you a boost midway through your day. And remember to eat a balanced meal at dinner.

Portion sizes

Look closely at the portions on your plate—often those portions are at least double the recommended serving sizes. Here are a few tips:

1. Use smaller plates. Our instinct is to fill a plate with food, which can be considerably more than we really need.

2. Occasionally measure your portions to find out how large a serving size is. A recipe itself is a good place to start. If there are four of you at the table and the dish serves six, you should have leftovers.

3. In restaurants, order half-portions when possible, or share a full portion with a friend.

4. Don't feel a need to finish your meal. Eat slowly, enjoy every bite and stop when you are full, not when the plate is empty.

> **Fruit and vegetable serving sizes**
>
> It's not hard to fit 5 to 10 servings of fruit and vegetables into your day. These examples represent one serving as outlined in *Canada's Food Guide to Healthy Eating*:
>
> 1 medium-sized fruit or vegetable (about the size of a tennis ball)
>
> 1 cup (250 mL) salad greens
>
> 1/2 cup (125 mL) fresh, frozen or canned fruits or vegetables
>
> 1/2 cup (125 mL) 100% fruit or vegetable juice
>
> 1/4 cup (60 mL) dried fruit

Variety

Eating a variety of foods enables you to enjoy different flavours and also provides you with a full range of vitamins and minerals. Choose wisely from the different food groups and look for healthy, appealing substitutes to your favourite, but not-so-healthy, treats. For example, a low-fat muffin can fulfill that urge for a doughnut, or a glass of low-fat chocolate milk will satisfy a craving for chocolate.

These small adjustments are simple, common sense habits that will make a big difference to your health and energy. Before you know it, you'll be reaching for healthier food without a second thought—and your body will thank you for it.

Canada's Food Guide to Healthy Eating

Canada's Food Guide to Healthy Eating outlines the healthy nutritional food choices available to us. The *Food Guide* stresses the need to eat a variety of foods from each food group in order to receive a full range of vitamins and minerals. Consider your age, lifestyle and calorie requirements when making your selections. For example, an active teenage boy will need a higher number of daily servings than an only moderately active 40-year-old woman.

Use the *Food Guide* (available online at Health Canada) to help you make healthy food choices, and look for healthy, low-fat, low-salt choices within each food group. For instance, an apple pie may fall into the category of a fruit serving, but unsweetened applesauce is a much better, low-fat alternative. Here are some other ideas for each food group:

Grain products (5 to 12 servings a day)
A single slice of bread or 3/4 cup (175 mL) of hot cereal constitutes 1 serving size. Try to choose whole grains because they contain more fibre and zinc than refined grain products. Look for cereals and pasta enriched with iron and B vitamins. Although cookies, cakes and croissants fall into this category, they aren't considered a smart choice, so save these treats as an occasional indulgence.

Vegetables and fruit (5 to 10 servings a day)
A half-cup (125 mL) of juice or a medium-sized carrot is all it takes to make up 1 serving in this important category. Colour is key here: Dark green, leafy vegetables and orange vegetables and fruit are all rich in vitamin A and folacin. Vividly coloured fruits and vegetables are higher in antioxidants and phytochemicals, and fruits like apples, strawberries and citrus offer soluble fibre— all valuable for reducing the risk of heart disease and some cancers. Canned produce contains the same amount of nutrients, but rinse the vegetables to reduce the salt and choose fruit that has been canned in its own juices.

Milk products (Daily: children—2 to 3 servings; youth—3 to 4 servings; adults—2 to 4 servings; pregnant and breast-feeding women—3 to 4 servings)
One cup (250 mL) of milk or 3/4 cup (175 mL) of yogurt constitutes 1 serving. Look for lower-fat or fat-free alternatives in this category. The fat content in milk will not change the amount of vitamins A and D, but keep in mind that milk products like yogurt and cheese don't have added vitamin D.

Meat and alternatives (2 to 3 servings a day)
Pay attention to serving size and fat content: one serving of cooked meat or fish weighs only 2 to 3 ounces (57 to 85 g)—about the size of a deck of cards. Red meat is a better source of iron than poultry, but choose lean cuts, if possible. As an alternative, legumes (peas, beans and lentils) provide significant amounts of starch and fibre. The *Food Guide* recommends you try to include legumes in your menu plan at least once or twice a week.

Other foods
The *Food Guide* also recognizes foods that fall outside the four main food groups. Things like condiments, cooking oils, candy, snack foods, soft drinks and alcohol can be high in fat, salt or sugar. These should only be an occasional choice.

Making Healthier Choices

Many health organizations agree that eating the right foods can help reduce the risk of heart attacks, stroke, hypertension and some forms of cancer. It begins with finding the right balance of food choices that works for you and your family. Include a wide variety of foods and remember:

Follow *Canada's Food Guide to Healthy Eating*
Choose more frequently from the first two food groups: whole-grain products and enriched cereals, and colourful selections of fruit and vegetables. Fruit and vegetables, in particular, play a key role in fighting heart disease, hypertension and some cancers because they are naturally rich in antioxidants, phytochemicals and fibre, and low in fat and sodium.

Reduce the fat
Whenever possible, choose low-fat dairy products, leaner cuts of meat and foods prepared with little or no cooking oil. Remove skin from poultry and limit your use of gravies and other high-fat sauces. Think about adding legumes once or twice to the weekly menu as an alternative to a meat serving, and try to minimize consumption of high-fat snack foods whenever possible.

Watch the salt
Avoid processed foods such as pre-packaged dinners, mixes and soups when you can. Add salt to your food at the table and not while cooking or, better yet, flavour with herbs and spices instead. And make cured meat, such as bacon, ham and salami, only an occasional choice.

You'll notice none of the recommendations include eliminating any one kind of food. The primary goal of healthy eating is to create good eating habits you can live with. Beyond these key points, *Canada's Food Guide to Healthy Eating* also suggests including regular physical activity as part of your daily schedule. Start making healthier choices today and the benefits will last a lifetime.

10

Apricot Breakfast Drink

Golden and creamy, with a frothy layer on top. A satisfying start to your day!

Can of apricot halves in light syrup (with syrup)	14 oz.	398 mL
Ice cubes	16	16
Milk	1 cup	250 mL
Low-fat plain yogurt	1/2 cup	125 mL
Liquid honey	2 tbsp.	30 mL
Ground nutmeg	1/8 tsp.	0.5 mL

Process all 6 ingredients in blender until smooth. Makes about 5 cups (1.25 L). Pour into 3 large glasses. Serves 3.

1 serving: 173 Calories; 1.1 g Total Fat (0.3 g Mono, 0.1 g Poly, 0.6 g Sat); 4 mg Cholesterol; 38 g Carbohydrate; 1 g Fibre; 6 g Protein; 79 mg Sodium

Pictured on page 71.

Cherry Almond Delight

A thick, sweet, lavender-coloured drink that might remind you of Cherries Jubilee. Add more milk to thin, if desired.

Can of pitted Bing cherries in heavy syrup (with syrup), chilled	14 oz.	398 mL
Light vanilla ice cream	1 cup	250 mL
Milk	3/4 cup	175 mL
Almond flavouring	1/8 tsp.	0.5 mL
Ground cinnamon (optional)	1/4 tsp.	1 mL

Process all 5 ingredients in blender until smooth. Makes about 3 3/4 cups (925 mL). Pour into 2 chilled large glasses. Serves 2.

1 serving: 360 Calories; 9 g Total Fat (2.6 g Mono, 0.4 g Poly, 5.5 g Sat); 35 mg Cholesterol; 67 g Carbohydrate; 2 g Fibre; 7 g Protein; 111 mg Sodium

Pictured on page 17.

 tip Instead of buying yogurt and fruit combinations that often contain added sugar, cut up and stir fresh fruit into low-fat plain yogurt for a lower calorie option.

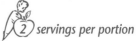

Banana Smoothie

This creamy, sunny yellow drink is a great way to say "Good morning."

Can of sliced peaches in pear juice (with syrup)	14 oz.	398 mL
Vanilla frozen yogurt	1 cup	250 mL
Overripe medium banana, cut up	1	1
Wheat germ	1 tbsp.	15 mL
Ice cubes	4	4

Process all 5 ingredients in blender until smooth. Makes about 3 1/2 cups (875 mL). Pour into 2 chilled large glasses. Serves 2.

1 serving: 319 Calories; 6.4 g Total Fat (1.7 g Mono, 0.5 g Poly, 3.8 g Sat); 10 mg Cholesterol; 64 g Carbohydrate; 4 g Fibre; 7 g Protein; 71 mg Sodium

BANANA SLUSHY: Peel and cut banana into 2 inch (5 cm) pieces. Freeze until firm (see Tip, below). Process with other ingredients as directed.

Creamy Raspberry Cooler

Pink, thick and creamy. Delightfully refreshing any time of day.

Container of frozen raspberries in syrup, partially thawed (see Note)	15 oz.	425 g
Low-fat raspberry yogurt	3/4 cup	175 mL
Milk	1/2 cup	125 mL

Process all 3 ingredients in blender until smooth. Makes about 3 1/4 cups (800 mL). Pour into 2 large glasses. Serves 2.

1 serving: 306 Calories; 1.2 g Total Fat (0.3 g Mono, 0.2 g Poly, 0.6 g Sat); 5 mg Cholesterol; 69 g Carbohydrate; 9 g Fibre; 8 g Protein; 103 mg Sodium

Pictured on page 125 and on back cover.

Note: If you prefer a seedless cooler, thaw raspberries completely and press through sieve into medium bowl to remove seeds. Cooler will not be as thick.

 Overripe bananas provide rich flavour to beverages. To use, peel and cut bananas into 2 inch (5 cm) pieces. Arrange in single layer in ungreased 9 x 13 inch (22 x 33 cm) pan. Freeze until firm. Store in resealable freezer bag. Use 4 pieces for 1 medium banana.

Peach Cooler

Cool and fizzy—just peachy any time!

Canned sliced peaches in pear juice, drained	1/2 cup	125 mL
Ice cubes	16	16
Club soda (or lemon lime soft drink)	1 cup	250 mL
White grape juice	1 cup	250 mL

Process peaches in blender until smooth. Spoon into 2 large glasses. Put 8 ice cubes in each glass.

Slowly add 1/2 cup (125 mL) each club soda and grape juice to each glass. Stir gently. Makes about 2 1/3 cups (575 mL). Serves 2.

1 serving: 97 Calories; 0.2 g Total Fat (0 g Mono, 0.1 g Poly, 0 g Sat); 0 mg Cholesterol; 24 g Carbohydrate; 1 g Fibre; 1 g Protein; 33 mg Sodium

2 servings per portion

Strawberry Lemonade

This frothy pink drink tends to separate quickly, but it's so good it won't last long enough to tell!

Pink lemonade	2 cups	500 mL
Fresh strawberries	2 cups	500 mL
Ice		
Fresh strawberries, for garnish	2	2

Process lemonade and strawberries in blender until smooth. Makes about 3 3/4 cups (925 mL).

Put ice into 2 large glasses. Add strawberry mixture. Garnish each with a fresh strawberry. Serves 2.

1 serving: 150 Calories; 0.6 g Total Fat (0.1 g Mono, 0.3 g Poly, 0.1 g Sat); 0 mg Cholesterol; 38 g Carbohydrate; 3 g Fibre; 1 g Protein; 9 mg Sodium

Pictured on page 17.

Apricot Lassi

Start or end your day with this sweet, tangy lassi. An easy-to-make refreshment—morning, noon or night.

Can of apricot halves in light syrup (with syrup)	14 oz.	398 mL
Low-fat plain yogurt	1 cup	250 mL
Milk	1/2 cup	125 mL
Liquid honey	3 tbsp.	50 mL
Ground almonds	3 tbsp.	50 mL
Ground cinnamon	1/8 tsp.	0.5 mL
Ice cubes	4	4

Process all 7 ingredients in blender until smooth. Makes about 3 3/4 cups (925 mL). Pour into 2 large glasses. Serves 2.

1 serving: 333 Calories; 4.1 g Total Fat (2.4 g Mono, 0.7 g Poly, 0.8 g Sat); 5 mg Cholesterol; 68 g Carbohydrate; 2 g Fibre; 11 g Protein; 133 mg Sodium

Banana Melon Shake

Frothy and refreshing. Nutmeg adds the perfect touch.

Milk	2 cups	500 mL
Chopped cantaloupe	1 cup	250 mL
Frozen overripe medium banana (see Tip, page 12)	1	1
Light vanilla ice cream	1/2 cup	125 mL
Ground nutmeg	1/8 tsp.	0.5 mL

Process all 5 ingredients in blender until smooth. Makes about 4 cups (1 L). Pour into 4 chilled medium glasses. Serves 4.

1 serving: 131 Calories; 3.6 g Total Fat (1 g Mono, 0.2 g Poly, 2.1 g Sat); 13 mg Cholesterol; 21 g Carbohydrate; 1 g Fibre; 6 g Protein; 83 mg Sodium

Yogurt Mango Shake

Lime and mango offer a taste of the tropics. Great for sunny days or when you need an armchair vacation.

Can of sliced mango in syrup (with syrup)	14 oz.	398 mL
Vanilla frozen yogurt	1 cup	250 mL
Milk	3/4 cup	175 mL
Grated lime zest	1/2 tsp.	2 mL
Ice cubes	4	4

Process all 5 ingredients in blender until smooth. Makes about 3 1/2 cups (875 mL). Pour into 2 large glasses. Serves 2.

1 serving: 367 Calories; 7 g Total Fat (2 g Mono, 0.3 g Poly, 4.3 g Sat); 14 mg Cholesterol; 73 g Carbohydrate; 2 g Fibre; 8 g Protein; 153 mg Sodium

Pictured on page 17.

Tropical Soy Shake

Shake up your day with this pineapple smoothie.

Can of pineapple chunks (with juice)	14 oz.	398 mL
Soy milk	1 cup	250 mL
Frozen overripe medium banana (see Tip, page 12)	1	1
Ice cubes	4	4
Ground nutmeg, sprinkle (optional)		

Process all 5 ingredients in blender until smooth. Makes about 4 cups (1 L). Pour into 4 medium glasses. Serves 4.

1 serving: 110 Calories; 1.4 g Total Fat (0.2 g Mono, 0.6 g Poly, 0.2 g Sat); 0 mg Cholesterol; 24 g Carbohydrate; 2 g Fibre; 2 g Protein; 9 mg Sodium

Chocolate Peach Smoothie

An irresistible combination that will jump-start your day.

Can of sliced peaches in pear juice (with juice)	14 oz.	398 mL
Milk	1 cup	250 mL
Low-fat vanilla yogurt	1/3 cup	75 mL
Chocolate syrup	2 tbsp.	30 mL

Process all 4 ingredients in blender until smooth. Makes about 3 1/2 cups (875 mL). Pour into 2 large glasses. Serves 2.

1 serving: 227 Calories; 2.4 g Total Fat (0.7 g Mono, 0.1 g Poly, 1.5 g Sat); 7 mg Cholesterol; 48 g Carbohydrate; 2 g Fibre; 8 g Protein; 116 mg Sodium

Dairy-Free Berry Smoothie

Just a little different, but very berry good!

Rice milk (such as Rice Dream)	1 1/2 cups	375 mL
Frozen mixed berries	1 cup	250 mL
Blueberry syrup (or liquid honey)	2 tbsp.	30 mL

Process all 3 ingredients in blender until smooth. Makes about 2 1/4 cups (550 mL). Pour into 2 medium glasses. Serves 2.

1 serving: 191 Calories; 1.9 g Total Fat (1.2 g Mono, 0.3 g Poly, 0.2 g Sat); 0 mg Cholesterol; 45 g Carbohydrate; 3 g Fibre; 1 g Protein; 87 mg Sodium

1. Yogurt Mango Shake, page 15
2. Cherry Almond Delight, page 11
3. Strawberry Lemonade, page 13

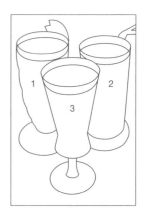

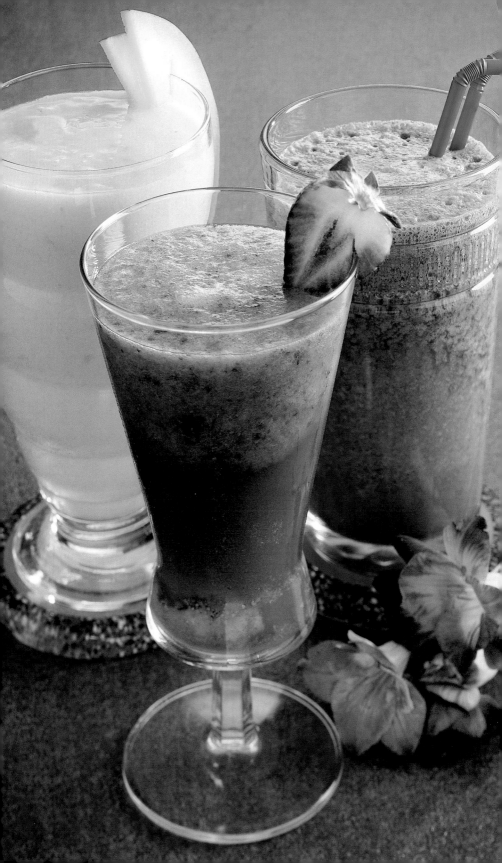

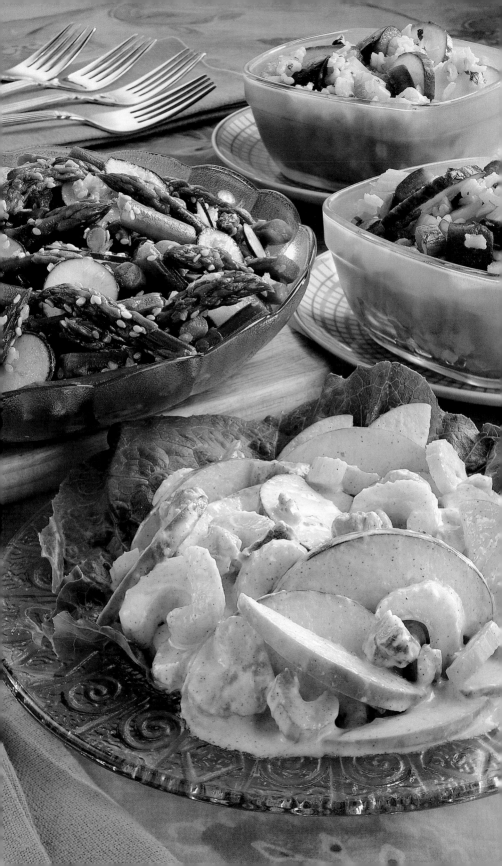

Orange Poppy Seed Coleslaw

Crisp and crunchy with a tasty orange dressing. It's worth a try!

Shredded red cabbage, lightly packed	3 cups	750 mL
Thinly sliced celery	1/2 cup	125 mL
Medium orange, segmented and cut into bite-size pieces	1	1
Green onions, chopped	4	4
ORANGE POPPY SEED DRESSING		
Orange juice	2 tbsp.	30 mL
Liquid honey	1 tbsp.	15 mL
Dijon mustard	1 tbsp.	15 mL
Olive (or cooking) oil	1 tbsp.	15 mL
Poppy seeds	2 tsp.	5 mL
Pepper	1/4 tsp.	1 mL

Put first 4 ingredients into large bowl. Toss gently.

Orange Poppy Seed Dressing: Combine all 6 ingredients in jar with tight-fitting lid. Shake well. Makes about 1/3 cup (75 mL) dressing. Drizzle over salad. Toss gently. Serves 6.

1 serving: 59 Calories; 3 g Total Fat (1.8 g Mono, 0.7 g Poly, 0.4 g Sat); 0 mg Cholesterol; 8 g Carbohydrate; 1 g Fibre; 1 g Protein; 49 mg Sodium

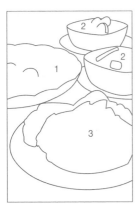

1. Asparagus and Radish Salad, page 24
2. Veggie Rice Salad, page 29
3. Apple Celery Salad, page 28

Props courtesy of: Canhome Global

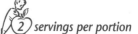

Bean, Ham and Potato Salad

A well-rounded salad with a zesty dressing that's a change from the ordinary.
Fabulously full of flavour!

Red baby potatoes, quartered	1 lb.	454 g
Boiling water		
Fresh (or frozen) whole green beans	2 cups	500 mL
Boiling water		
Ice water		
Cherry (or grape) tomatoes, halved	20	20
Low-fat deli ham, cut into thin strips	6 oz.	170 g
Chopped red onion	1/2 cup	125 mL
MUSTARD DRESSING		
Orange juice	3 tbsp.	50 mL
Finely chopped gherkin (or dill pickle)	2 tbsp.	30 mL
Light sour cream	2 tbsp.	30 mL
Dijon mustard (with whole seeds)	1 tbsp.	15 mL
Ground cumin	1/2 tsp.	2 mL
Garlic clove, minced	1	1
(or 1/4 tsp., 1 mL, powder)		

Cook potato in boiling water in medium saucepan until just tender. Drain. Cool.

Cook green beans in boiling water in medium saucepan for about 5 minutes until bright green. Drain. Immediately plunge into ice water in medium bowl. Let stand for about 10 minutes until cold. Drain well. Cut green beans into 2 inch (5 cm) pieces.

Combine next 3 ingredients in large bowl. Add potato and green beans. Toss gently.

Mustard Dressing: Combine all 6 ingredients in jar with tight-fitting lid. Shake well. Makes about 1/2 cup (125 mL) dressing. Drizzle over salad. Toss gently. Serves 6.

1 serving: 163 Calories; 4.3 g Total Fat (2 g Mono, 0.6 g Poly, 1.5 g Sat); 17 mg Cholesterol; 24 g Carbohydrate; 3 g Fibre; 9 g Protein; 431 mg Sodium

Pictured on page 53.

Shell Shrimp Salad

Mild creamy dressing coats peas and pasta—a perfect pair with succulent shrimp.

Tiny shell pasta	1 1/2 cups	375 mL
Boiling water	8 cups	2 L
Salt	1 tsp.	5 mL
Frozen peas	3 cups	750 mL
Cooked salad shrimp	6 oz.	170 g
Diced celery	1/2 cup	125 mL
Finely chopped red onion	2 tbsp.	30 mL
Large hard-cooked eggs, chopped	3	3
HORSERADISH DRESSING		
Light mayonnaise	2/3 cup	150 mL
Ketchup	2 tbsp.	30 mL
Milk	1 tbsp.	15 mL
Granulated sugar	1 tsp.	5 mL
Creamed horseradish	1 tsp.	5 mL
Onion powder	1/4 tsp.	1 mL
Chopped or torn romaine lettuce, lightly packed	6 cups	1.5 L

Cook pasta in boiling water and salt in large uncovered pot or Dutch oven for 6 to 8 minutes, stirring occasionally, until tender but firm. Add peas during last 3 minutes of cooking time. Drain. Rinse with cold water. Drain well. Transfer to large bowl.

Add next 4 ingredients. Toss gently.

Horseradish Dressing: Combine first 6 ingredients in small bowl. Makes about 1 cup (250 mL) dressing. Drizzle over pasta mixture. Toss gently.

Spread lettuce evenly on large serving platter. Spoon pasta mixture onto lettuce. Serves 6.

1 serving: 319 Calories; 12.3 g Total Fat (6.2 g Mono, 3.4 g Poly, 1.6 g Sat); 163 mg Cholesterol; 35 g Carbohydrate; 2 g Fibre; 17 g Protein; 362 mg Sodium

Ambrosia Fruit Salad

A classic combination that's always a favourite. Use coloured marshmallows for a rainbow effect the kids will enjoy.

Low-fat peach yogurt	1 cup	250 mL
Light sour cream	1/2 cup	125 mL
Can of fruit cocktail, drained	14 oz.	398 mL
Can of mandarin orange segments, drained	10 oz.	284 mL
Pineapple tidbits, drained	1 cup	250 mL
Miniature marshmallows	1 cup	250 mL
Medium sweetened coconut, toasted (see Tip, page 47)	1/4 cup	60 mL

Combine yogurt and sour cream in large bowl. Add next 4 ingredients. Stir gently.

Sprinkle with coconut. Serves 4.

1 serving: 199 Calories; 4 g Total Fat (1.4 g Mono, 0.2 g Poly, 4.2 g Sat); 8 mg Cholesterol; 39 g Carbohydrate; 2 g Fibre; 5 g Protein; 82 mg Sodium

Beet Coleslaw

A little different from the ordinary, but sure to be a hit! Refreshing dill and tangy lemon make a memorable dressing.

ZESTY DILL DRESSING		
Light mayonnaise	1/2 cup	125 mL
Lemon juice	1 tbsp.	15 mL
Chopped fresh dill (or 1/4 tsp., 1 mL, dried)	1 tsp.	5 mL
Dry mustard	1/2 tsp.	2 mL
Shredded green cabbage, lightly packed	2 cups	500 mL
Can of sliced beets, drained, chopped	14 oz.	398 mL
1% cottage cheese	1 cup	250 mL
Shredded red cabbage, lightly packed	1 cup	250 mL

(continued on next page)

Zesty Dill Dressing: Combine first 4 ingredients in small bowl. Makes about 1/2 cup (125 mL) dressing.

Put remaining 4 ingredients into large bowl. Drizzle with dressing. Toss well. Serves 8.

1 serving: 87 Calories; 5.3 g Total Fat (3 g Mono, 1.5 g Poly, 0.5 g Sat); 1 mg Cholesterol; 6 g Carbohydrate; 1 g Fibre; 5 g Protein; 307 mg Sodium

Pictured on page 126.

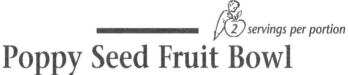 *servings per portion*

Poppy Seed Fruit Bowl

Avocado adds a nice touch to an array of juicy fruits coated in creamy dressing. Use any seasonal fruit.

POPPY SEED DRESSING

Low-fat vanilla (or plain) yogurt	1 cup	250 mL
Liquid honey	1 tbsp.	15 mL
Lemon juice	2 tsp.	10 mL
Poppy seeds	2 tsp.	10 mL
Ground ginger	1/4 tsp.	1 mL
Mandarin oranges, segmented	8	8
Red medium grapefruits, segmented and cut into bite-size pieces	4	4
Medium avocados, cut into 1/2 inch (12 mm) pieces	2	2
Seedless red grapes	1 cup	250 mL
Seedless green grapes	1 cup	250 mL

Poppy Seed Dressing: Combine first 5 ingredients in small bowl. Makes about 1 cup (250 mL) dressing.

Put remaining 5 ingredients into large bowl. Drizzle with dressing. Toss gently. Serves 10.

1 serving: 171 Calories; 7.2 g Total Fat (4.1 g Mono, 1 g Poly, 1.4 g Sat); 1 mg Cholesterol; 28 g Carbohydrate; 4 g Fibre; 3 g Protein; 20 mg Sodium

Pictured on page 125 and on back cover.

Asparagus and Radish Salad

Zesty lemon and mustard dressing adds the perfect punch to crisp asparagus.
Looks pretty with a sprinkling of sesame seeds.

Fresh asparagus, trimmed of tough ends and cut into 2 inch (5 cm) pieces	1 lb.	454 g
Boiling water		
Ice water		
Thinly sliced radish	1 cup	250 mL
Sesame seeds, toasted (see Tip, page 47)	2 tbsp.	30 mL
LEMON DRESSING		
Olive (or cooking) oil	2 tbsp.	30 mL
Finely chopped shallots (or green onion)	2 tbsp.	30 mL
White wine vinegar	1 tbsp.	15 mL
Lemon juice	1 tbsp.	15 mL
Liquid honey	2 tsp.	10 mL
Dijon mustard	1 tsp.	5 mL
Garlic clove, minced (or 1/4 tsp., 1 mL, powder)	1	1
Grated lemon zest	1/4 tsp.	1 mL
Pepper, sprinkle		

Cook asparagus in boiling water in large saucepan for about 5 minutes until bright green. Drain. Immediately plunge into ice water in large bowl. Let stand for about 10 minutes until cold. Drain well. Transfer to medium bowl.

Add radish and sesame seeds. Toss.

Lemon Dressing: Combine all 9 ingredients in jar with tight-fitting lid. Shake well. Makes about 1/3 cup (75 mL) dressing. Drizzle over salad. Toss well. Serves 4.

1 serving: 139 Calories; 9.7 g Total Fat (6.1 g Mono, 1.7 g Poly, 1.3 g Sat); 0 mg Cholesterol; 12 g Carbohydrate; 3 g Fibre; 4 g Protein; 12 mg Sodium

Pictured on page 18.

Mushroom Cranberry Salad

A delicious blend of both sweet and tart. Using a variety of mushrooms, such as oyster, brown and white, adds interest. Try a mixture of green and red leaf lettuce for a colourful contrast.

Olive (or cooking) oil	1 tbsp.	15 mL
Sliced fresh mushrooms (your favourite)	4 cups	1 L
Red wine vinegar	1 tbsp.	15 mL
Liquid honey	1 tbsp.	15 mL
Chopped or torn green leaf lettuce, lightly packed	5 cups	1.25 L
Crumbled light feta cheese	3/4 cup	175 mL
CRANBERRY DRESSING		
Olive (or cooking) oil	3 tbsp.	50 mL
Jellied cranberry sauce, warmed	3 tbsp.	50 mL
Red wine vinegar	2 tbsp.	30 mL

Heat olive oil in large frying pan on medium. Add mushrooms. Cook for 5 to 10 minutes, stirring often, until mushrooms are softened.

Add vinegar and honey. Heat and stir for about 1 minute until mushrooms are coated and liquid is evaporated. Transfer to large bowl. Cool slightly.

Add lettuce and cheese. Toss gently.

Cranberry Dressing: Combine all 3 ingredients in jar with tight-fitting lid. Shake well. Makes about 1/2 cup (125 mL) dressing. Drizzle over salad. Toss gently. Serves 8.

1 serving: 133 Calories; 10.2 g Total Fat (5.7 g Mono, 0.8 g Poly, 3.1 g Sat); 13 mg Cholesterol; 9 g Carbohydrate; 1 g Fibre; 3 g Protein; 169 mg Sodium

 tip Reduce fat in your diet by using less dressing or a low-fat dressing on your salad. Measure your salad dressing rather than pouring it straight from the bottle.

Warm Mushroom Salad

Lots of great flavours in this salad. Perfect for mushroom fans!

Red wine vinegar	1 tbsp.	15 mL
Liquid honey, warmed	1 tbsp.	15 mL
Garlic cloves, minced	2	2
(or 1/2 tsp., 2 mL, powder)		
Small brown mushrooms	2 cups	500 mL
Small white mushrooms	2 cups	500 mL
Mixed salad greens, lightly packed	4 cups	1 L
Jar of roasted red peppers, drained,	12 oz.	340 mL
blotted dry, cut into thin strips		
Fresh bean sprouts	1 cup	250 mL
Basil pesto	1 tbsp.	15 mL
Red wine vinegar	1 tbsp.	15 mL

Combine first 3 ingredients in large bowl. Add brown and white mushrooms. Toss until coated. Spread in single layer in greased baking sheet with sides. Bake in 450°F (230°C) oven for about 10 minutes, stirring once, until mushrooms start to soften. Return to same large bowl.

Add next 3 ingredients. Toss.

Combine pesto and second amount of vinegar in small bowl. Drizzle over salad. Toss well. Serves 8.

1 serving: 48 Calories; 1 g Total Fat (0.4 g Mono, 0.2 g Poly, 0.1 g Sat); 0 mg Cholesterol; 9 g Carbohydrate; 2 g Fibre; 3 g Protein; 66 mg Sodium

Pictured on page 54.

Spinach and Raspberry Salad

An imaginative combination of fruit and vegetables. Scrumptious with grilled steak.

Fresh spinach, stems removed,	5 cups	1.25 L
lightly packed		
Fresh raspberries	1 cup	250 mL
Thinly sliced fresh white mushrooms	1 cup	250 mL
Sliced natural almonds, toasted	1/3 cup	75 mL
(see Tip, page 47)		

(continued on next page)

RASPBERRY VINAIGRETTE

Fresh raspberries	1/4 cup	60 mL
Raspberry (or red wine) vinegar	2 tbsp.	30 mL
Olive (or cooking) oil	1 tbsp.	15 mL
Granulated sugar	1 tsp.	5 mL
Dijon mustard	1 tsp.	5 mL
Pepper	1/4 tsp.	1 mL

Put first 4 ingredients into large bowl. Toss gently.

Raspberry Vinaigrette: Process all 6 ingredients in blender or food processor until smooth. Makes about 1/2 cup (125 mL) dressing. Drizzle over salad. Toss gently. Serves 6.

1 serving: 84 Calories; 5.9 g Total Fat (3.8 g Mono, 1.1 g Poly, 0.7 g Sat); 0 mg Cholesterol; 7 g Carbohydrate; 3 g Fibre; 3 g Protein; 37 mg Sodium

---

Minted Pea Salad

A salad that's sure to "pea-lease!" Great with your favourite barbecue meal.

Sugar snap peas, trimmed	2 cups	500 mL
Snow peas, trimmed	2 cups	500 mL
Boiling water		
Ice water		
Pea sprouts	1 cup	250 mL
MINT DRESSING		
Cooking oil	3 tbsp.	50 mL
Lemon juice	2 tbsp.	30 mL
Mint jelly	1 tbsp.	15 mL
Dijon mustard (with whole seeds)	1 tbsp.	15 mL
Granulated sugar	1 tsp.	5 mL

Cook sugar snap and snow peas in boiling water in medium saucepan for about 5 minutes until bright green. Drain. Immediately plunge into ice water in medium bowl. Let stand for about 10 minutes until cold. Drain well. Blot dry with paper towels. Transfer to large bowl.

Add pea sprouts. Toss.

Mint Dressing: Combine all 5 ingredients in jar with tight-fitting lid. Shake well. Makes about 1/2 cup (125 mL) dressing. Drizzle over salad. Toss well. Serves 6.

1 serving: 120 Calories; 7.3 g Total Fat (4.1 g Mono, 2.3 g Poly, 0.6 g Sat); 0 mg Cholesterol; 11 g Carbohydrate; 2 g Fibre; 3 g Protein; 46 mg Sodium

Cottage Cheese Crunch

A tasty way to dress up cottage cheese for lunch.

Tart unpeeled medium cooking apples (such as Granny Smith), diced,	2	2
1% cottage cheese	1 cup	250 mL
Shredded cabbage, lightly packed	1 cup	250 mL
Salted roasted sunflower seeds	3 tbsp.	50 mL
Chopped pecans, toasted (see Tip, page 47)	3 tbsp.	50 mL
Light mayonnaise	2 tbsp.	30 mL
Pepper	1/4 tsp.	1 mL

Put all 7 ingredients into large bowl. Toss gently. Serves 4.

1 serving: 167 Calories; 9.9 g Total Fat (4.5 g Mono, 3.7 g Poly, 1.2 g Sat); 3 mg Cholesterol; 11 g Carbohydrate; 2 g Fibre; 10 g Protein; 351 mg Sodium

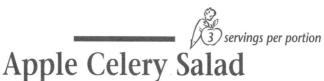 *servings per portion*

Apple Celery Salad

A Waldorf-style salad full of sweet apple, crisp celery and crunchy walnuts—all coated with a creamy cinnamon dressing.

YOGURT CINNAMON DRESSING		
Low-fat plain yogurt	1 cup	250 mL
Lemon juice	1 tbsp.	15 mL
Liquid honey	1 tbsp.	15 mL
Ground cinnamon	1/4 tsp.	1 mL
Medium unpeeled cooking apples (such as McIntosh), quartered and sliced	3	3
Thinly sliced celery	1 cup	250 mL
Chopped walnuts, toasted (see Tip, page 47)	1/4 cup	60 mL
Romaine (or iceberg) lettuce leaves	4	4

Yogurt Cinnamon Dressing: Combine first 4 ingredients in large bowl. Makes about 1 cup (250 mL) dressing.

Add next 3 ingredients. Stir until coated.

Place 1 lettuce leaf on each of 4 plates. Spoon apple mixture onto each leaf. Serves 4.

(continued on next page)

Salads

1 serving: 177 Calories; 6.2 g Total Fat (1.4 g Mono, 3.3 g Poly, 1 g Sat); 4 mg Cholesterol; 28 g Carbohydrate; 3 g Fibre; 6 g Protein; 74 mg Sodium

Pictured on page 18.

Veggie Rice Salad

A fresh-tasting salad with an Asian flair. Fresh herbs add lots of colour.

Cooked long grain brown rice (about 2/3 cup, 150 mL, uncooked)	2 cups	500 mL
Thinly sliced English cucumber (with peel)	1 cup	250 mL
Chopped red pepper	1 cup	250 mL
Chopped celery	1 cup	250 mL
Can of sliced water chestnuts, drained	8 oz.	227 mL
Chopped green onion	1/3 cup	75 mL
LIME HERB DRESSING		
Lime juice	3 tbsp.	50 mL
Chopped fresh cilantro or parsley	2 tbsp.	30 mL
Chopped fresh mint leaves	2 tbsp.	30 mL
Sweet chili sauce	1 tbsp.	15 mL
Cooking oil	1 tbsp.	15 mL
Fish sauce	1/2 tsp.	2 mL
Garlic clove, minced (or 1/4 tsp., 1 mL, powder)	1	1

Put first 6 ingredients into large bowl. Toss.

Lime Herb Dressing: Combine all 7 ingredients in jar with tight-fitting lid. Shake well. Makes about 1/3 cup (75 mL) dressing. Drizzle over salad. Toss well. Serves 6.

1 serving: 135 Calories; 3.1 g Total Fat (1.6 g Mono, 1 g Poly, 0.3 g Sat); 0 mg Cholesterol; 25 g Carbohydrate; 3 g Fibre; 3 g Protein; 95 mg Sodium

Pictured on page 18.

Paré Pointer

The computer programmer? He went data-way.

Tofu Spinach Salad

An Asian-inspired salad topped with crunchy fried noodles.

Rice stick noodles	2 oz.	57g
Cooking oil, for deep-frying		
Fresh spinach, stems removed, lightly packed	5 cups	1.25 L
Thinly sliced snow peas	1 1/3 cups	325 mL
Grated carrot	2/3 cup	150 mL
Coarsely chopped salted peanuts	1/2 cup	125 mL
Peanut (or cooking) oil	2 tsp.	10 mL
Package of firm tofu, drained, cut into 1/2 inch (12 mm) cubes	12 1/4 oz.	350 g
Low-sodium soy sauce	1 tbsp.	15 mL
Liquid honey	1 tbsp.	15 mL
GINGER DRESSING		
Peanut (or cooking) oil	1/4 cup	60 mL
Rice vinegar	2 tbsp.	30 mL
Liquid honey	2 tbsp.	30 mL
Sweet chili sauce	1 tbsp.	15 mL
Finely grated ginger root (or 1/4 tsp., 1 mL, ground)	1 tsp.	5 mL
Dried crushed chilies	1/2 tsp.	2 mL
Pepper	1/8 tsp.	0.5 mL

Separate noodles slightly. Deep-fry in hot (375°F, 190°C) cooking oil for about 1 minute until puffed. Remove with slotted spoon to paper towels to drain.

Put next 4 ingredients into large bowl. Toss. Set aside.

Heat peanut oil in large frying pan on medium. Add tofu. Cook for about 5 minutes, stirring often, until golden.

Add soy sauce and honey. Stir until coated. Add to spinach mixture. Toss gently.

Ginger Dressing: Combine all 7 ingredients in jar with tight-fitting lid. Shake well. Makes about 2/3 cup (150 mL) dressing. Drizzle over salad. Toss gently. Break up noodles. Sprinkle over top. Serves 8.

1 serving: 248 Calories; 17.2 g Total Fat (7.1 g Mono, 6.4 g Poly, 2.7 g Sat); 0 mg Cholesterol; 17 g Carbohydrate; 2 g Fibre; 10 g Protein; 180 mg Sodium

Salads

Warm Chicken Salad

A rich, colourful meal salad full of earthy flavour. A sure hit!

GARLIC AND HERB MARINADE

Balsamic vinegar	3 tbsp.	50 mL
Olive (or cooking) oil	2 tbsp.	30 mL
Chopped fresh oregano	1 tbsp.	15 mL
(or 3/4 tsp., 4 mL, dried)		
Garlic cloves, minced	2	2
(or 1/2 tsp., 2 mL, powder)		
Garlic and herb no-salt seasoning (such	1/2 tsp.	2 mL
as Mrs. Dash)		
Pepper	1/4 tsp.	1 mL
Boneless, skinless chicken breast halves,	1 lb.	454 g
chopped		
Cooked whole-wheat rotini (or other	3 cups	750 mL
spiral) pasta (about 2 1/4 cups,		
550 mL, uncooked)		
Sliced fresh brown (or white) mushrooms	2 cups	500 mL
Fresh spinach, stems removed,	2 cups	500 mL
lightly packed		
Crumbled light feta cheese	1 cup	250 mL
Roasted red peppers, drained, blotted	1/2 cup	125 mL
dry, cut into thin strips		

Garlic and Herb Marinade: Combine first 6 ingredients in medium bowl. Makes about 1/3 cup (75 mL) marinade. Add chicken. Stir until coated. Cover. Marinate in refrigerator for 20 minutes, stirring occasionally. Heat large frying pan on medium-high until hot. Add chicken with marinade. Cook for about 5 minutes, stirring occasionally, until chicken is no longer pink inside. Transfer to large bowl.

Add remaining 5 ingredients. Toss well. Serves 4.

1 serving: 457 Calories; 18.1 g Total Fat (7.5 g Mono, 1.6 g Poly, 7.4 g Sat); 84 mg Cholesterol; 35 g Carbohydrate; 5 g Fibre; 41 g Protein; 217 mg Sodium

Spiced Beef Soup

This rich broth seasoned with cumin and coriander provides a spicy taste of the East.
Serve with pappadums (PAH-pah-duhms), thin crackers made with lentil flour.

Cooking oil	1 tbsp.	15 mL
Stewing beef, cut into 1/2 inch (12 mm) pieces	3/4 lb.	340 g
Cooking oil	2 tsp.	10 mL
Chopped onion	1 1/2 cups	375 mL
Ground cumin	2 tsp.	10 mL
Ground coriander	2 tsp.	10 mL
Ground ginger	1 tsp.	5 mL
Dried crushed chilies	1 tsp.	5 mL
Can of diced tomatoes (with juice)	28 oz.	796 mL
Low-sodium prepared beef broth	4 cups	1 L
Can of chickpeas (garbanzo beans), rinsed and drained	19 oz.	540 mL
Medium zucchini (with peel), chopped	1	1
Chopped fresh mint leaves (or 1 1/2 tsp., 7 mL, dried)	2 tbsp.	30 mL
Liquid honey	2 tsp.	10 mL
Grated lemon zest	1 tsp.	5 mL

Heat first amount of cooking oil in large pot or Dutch oven on medium-high. Add beef. Cook for 5 to 10 minutes, stirring occasionally, until browned. Transfer to large bowl. Cover to keep warm.

Heat second amount of cooking oil in same large pot on medium. Add onion. Cook for 5 to 10 minutes, stirring often, until softened.

Add next 4 ingredients. Heat and stir for about 1 minute until fragrant.

Add beef, tomatoes and broth. Stir. Bring to a boil on medium-high. Reduce heat to medium-low. Cover. Simmer for 20 minutes, stirring occasionally.

Add chickpeas. Stir. Cover. Simmer for about 20 minutes until beef is very tender.

Add remaining 4 ingredients. Stir. Cook, uncovered, on medium for about 5 minutes until zucchini is tender. Serves 8.

1 serving: 200 Calories; 7.9 g Total Fat (3.5 g Mono, 1.5 g Poly, 1.8 g Sat); 24 mg Cholesterol; 19 g Carbohydrate; 3 g Fibre; 15 g Protein; 605 mg Sodium

Pictured on page 35.

Thai-Style Pork Soup

Spicy curry heats up this hearty soup. A great starter for an Asian meal.

Cooking oil	1 tbsp.	15 mL
Pork tenderloin, trimmed of fat and cut into thin strips (see Tip, page 101)	1/2 lb.	225 g
Thai red curry paste	1 tbsp.	15 mL
Low-sodium prepared chicken broth	4 cups	1 L
Can of cut baby corn, drained	14 oz.	398 mL
Thinly sliced red pepper	1 cup	250 mL
Fish sauce	1 tsp.	5 mL
Brown sugar, packed	1 tsp.	5 mL
Fresh spinach, stems removed, lightly packed	2 cups	500 mL
Finely shredded fresh basil (or 1 1/2 tsp., 7 mL, dried)	2 tbsp.	30 mL
Lime juice	1 tbsp.	15 mL

Heat cooking oil in large pot or Dutch oven on medium-high. Add pork. Cook for about 5 minutes, stirring occasionally, until browned. Transfer to small bowl. Cover to keep warm.

Heat and stir curry paste in same large pot on medium for about 1 minute until fragrant.

Add next 5 ingredients. Stir. Bring to a boil on medium-high. Reduce heat to medium-low. Cover. Simmer for about 5 minutes until red pepper is softened.

Add pork and spinach. Stir. Simmer for about 2 minutes, stirring occasionally, until pork is heated through and spinach is wilted.

Add basil and lime juice. Stir. Serves 4.

1 serving: 199 Calories; 7.7 g Total Fat (3.9 g Mono, 1.8 g Poly, 1.2 g Sat); 35 mg Cholesterol; 17 g Carbohydrate; 3 g Fibre; 18 g Protein; 907 mg Sodium

Pictured on page 35.

Curried Squash Soup

Squash your worries about what to feed the family with this velvety-textured golden soup.

Cooking oil	2 tsp.	10 mL
Chopped onion	2 cups	500 mL
Curry powder	1 1/2 tbsp.	25 mL
Finely grated ginger root	2 tsp.	10 mL
(or 1/2 tsp., 2 mL, ground)		
Chopped butternut squash	7 cups	1.75 L
Low-sodium prepared chicken broth	6 cups	1.5 L
Light sour cream	1/4 cup	60 mL
Pepper	1/4 tsp.	1 mL

Heat cooking oil in large pot or Dutch oven on medium. Add onion. Cook for 5 to 10 minutes, stirring often, until softened.

Add curry powder and ginger. Heat and stir for about 1 minute until fragrant.

Add squash and broth. Bring to a boil. Reduce heat to medium-low. Cover. Simmer for about 30 minutes, stirring occasionally, until squash is softened. Remove from heat. Cool slightly. Carefully process with hand blender, or in blender in 2 batches, until smooth (see Safety Tip). Return to same large pot.

Add sour cream and pepper. Heat and stir on medium until heated through. Serves 8.

1 serving: 108 Calories; 2.1 g Total Fat (1 g Mono, 0.5 g Poly, 0.8 g Sat); 2 mg Cholesterol; 21 g Carbohydrate; 3 g Fibre; 4 g Protein; 489 mg Sodium

Safety Tip: Follow blender manufacturer's instructions for processing hot liquids.

1. Spiced Beef Soup, page 32
2. Cabbage Lover's Soup, page 37
3. Thai-Style Pork Soup, page 33

Props courtesy of: Cherison Enterprises Inc.
Danesco Inc.
Casa Bugatti

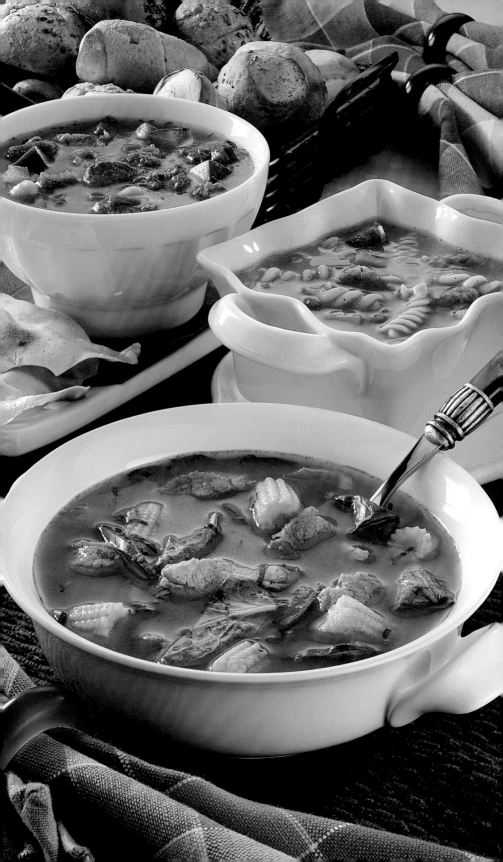

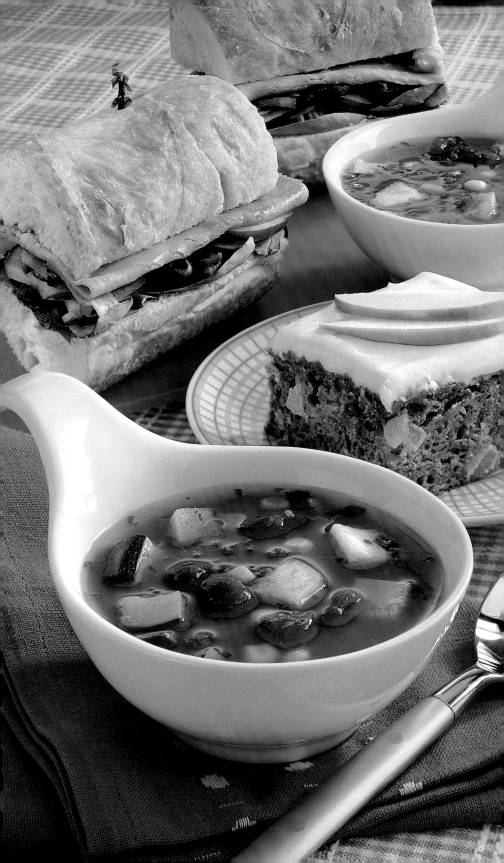

Cabbage Lover's Soup

Get your fill of cabbage with this Italian-style soup. Serve with crusty rolls.

Cooking oil	2 tsp.	10 mL
Chopped cabbage	4 cups	1 L
Thinly sliced leek (white part only)	1 cup	250 mL
Thinly sliced celery	1 cup	250 mL
Diced carrot	1 cup	250 mL
Prepared vegetable broth	8 cups	2 L
Can of diced tomatoes (with juice)	14 oz.	398 mL
Italian seasoning	1 tsp.	5 mL
Fusilli (or other spiral) pasta	1 cup	250 mL

Heat cooking oil in large pot or Dutch oven on medium-high. Add next 4 ingredients. Cook for 5 to 10 minutes, stirring occasionally, until vegetables start to soften.

Add next 3 ingredients. Stir. Bring to a boil. Reduce heat to medium-low. Cover. Simmer for 20 to 30 minutes until vegetables are tender-crisp.

Add pasta. Cook, uncovered, on medium-high for about 10 minutes, stirring occasionally, until pasta is tender but firm. Serves 8.

1 serving: 121 Calories; 2.3 g Total Fat (1 g Mono, 0.6 g Poly, 0.4 g Sat); 0 mg Cholesterol; 20 g Carbohydrate; 3 g Fibre; 6 g Protein; 995 mg Sodium

Pictured on page 35.

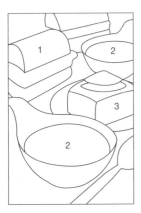

1. Mediterranean Sub, page 61
2. Tomato and Zucchini Soup, page 44
3. Apple Carrot Cake, page 141

Props courtesy of: Danesco Inc.

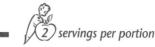

Cool and Zesty Soup

Garnish individual servings of this gazpacho-style soup with croutons or diced hard-cooked egg. Delightfully refreshing.

Medium tomatoes, peeled (see Tip, below) and coarsely chopped	5	5
English cucumber (with peel), coarsely chopped	1	1
Coarsely chopped red onion	2/3 cup	150 mL
Roasted red peppers, drained, blotted dry, chopped	1/3 cup	75 mL
Lemon juice	1 tbsp.	15 mL
Chopped fresh dill	1 tbsp.	15 mL
Balsamic vinegar	1/2 tbsp.	7 mL
Granulated sugar	3/4 tsp.	4 mL
Garlic cloves, minced	2	2
Hot pepper sauce	1/2 tsp.	2 mL
Pepper	1/8 tsp.	0.5 mL
Tomato juice	2 1/4 cups	560 mL

Put first 11 ingredients into food processor. Process with on/off motion until vegetables are finely chopped. Transfer 2 cups (500 mL) tomato mixture to large bowl. Process remaining mixture until almost smooth. Transfer to same large bowl.

Add tomato juice. Stir well. Cover. Chill for at least 3 hours until cold. Serves 8.

1 serving: 43 Calories; 0.4 g Total Fat (0.1 g Mono, 0.2 g Poly, 0.1 g Sat); 0 mg Cholesterol; 10 g Carbohydrate; 2 g Fibre; 2 g Protein; 289 mg Sodium

 To peel tomatoes, cut an X on the bottom, just through the skin. Plunge into boiling water for 30 seconds, then immediately into a bowl of ice water. Peel.

Chicken and Bacon Pea Soup

Back bacon adds rich, smoky flavour to this hearty soup.
Serve with salad or crusty bread.

Cooking oil	2 tsp.	10 mL
Chopped red pepper	1 cup	250 mL
Chopped green onion	1 cup	250 mL
Boneless, skinless chicken thighs, cut into 1/2 inch (12 mm) pieces	6 oz.	170 g
Chopped lean back (Canadian) bacon	1/3 cup	75 mL
Paprika	1/2 tsp.	2 mL
Pepper	1/2 tsp.	2 mL
All-purpose flour	2 tbsp.	30 mL
Milk	2 cups	500 mL
Low-sodium prepared chicken broth	2 cups	500 mL
Frozen peas	1 cup	250 mL
Light sour cream	2 tbsp.	30 mL

Heat cooking oil in large saucepan on medium. Add next 6 ingredients. Cook for 5 to 10 minutes, stirring occasionally, until chicken is no longer pink inside.

Add flour. Heat and stir for 1 minute.

Slowly add milk and broth, stirring constantly. Heat and stir until boiling and thickened. Reduce heat to medium-low. Simmer, uncovered, for 10 minutes, stirring occasionally.

Add peas and sour cream. Stir. Cover. Simmer for about 5 minutes, stirring occasionally, until peas are heated through. Serves 6.

1 serving: 149 Calories; 5 g Total Fat (2.1 g Mono, 1 g Poly, 1.7 g Sat); 33 mg Cholesterol; 13 g Carbohydrate; 2 g Fibre; 13 g Protein; 361 mg Sodium

Creamy Mushroom Soup

A long-time favourite you'll make again and again. Process longer if you prefer a smoother soup.

Sliced fresh mushrooms (your favourite)	6 cups	1.5 L
Cooking oil	2 tsp.	10 mL
Pepper, sprinkle		
Cooking oil	2 tsp.	10 mL
Chopped green onion	1/2 cup	125 mL
Garlic cloves, minced	2	2
All-purpose flour	3 tbsp.	50 mL
Low-sodium prepared chicken broth	2 cups	500 mL
Milk	2 cups	500 mL
Dry (or alcohol-free) white wine	1/4 cup	60 mL
Reduced-sodium chicken bouillon powder	2 tsp.	10 mL
Pepper	1/4 tsp.	1 mL
Ground thyme (optional)	1/8 tsp.	0.5 mL

Put mushrooms into medium bowl. Add first amount of cooking oil. Stir until coated. Spread in single layer in greased baking sheet with sides. Sprinkle with first amount of pepper. Bake in 400°F (205°C) oven for about 10 minutes until mushrooms are softened. Do not drain.

Heat second amount of cooking oil in large pot or Dutch oven on medium. Add green onion and garlic. Cook for about 5 minutes, stirring often, until green onion is softened.

Add flour. Heat and stir for 1 minute. Slowly add next 3 ingredients, stirring constantly until boiling and thickened.

Add mushrooms with liquid and remaining 3 ingredients. Heat and stir for 3 to 4 minutes. Reduce heat to medium-low. Cover. Simmer for 5 minutes. Remove from heat. Cool slightly. Carefully process in blender or food processor until mushrooms are finely chopped (see Safety Tip). Return to same large pot. Heat and stir on medium for about 5 minutes until heated through. Serves 6.

1 serving: 116 Calories; 4.5 g Total Fat (2.2 g Mono, 1.1 g Poly, 0.9 g Sat); 4 mg Cholesterol; 12 g Carbohydrate; 1 g Fibre; 6 g Protein; 392 mg Sodium

Safety Tip: Follow blender manufacturer's instructions for processing hot liquids.

Spicy Bean Soup

A marvelous Mexican-style soup that's perfect with tortilla chips.

Cooking oil	1 tsp.	5 mL
Chorizo sausages, casings removed, chopped	2	2
Cooking oil	1 tbsp.	15 mL
Finely chopped red onion	1 1/2 cups	375 mL
Finely chopped red pepper	1 1/2 cups	375 mL
Garlic cloves, minced (or 1/2 tsp., 2 mL, powder)	2	2
Chili powder	1 tbsp.	15 mL
Ground cumin	2 tsp.	10 mL
Low-sodium prepared chicken broth	6 cups	1.5 L
Can of diced tomatoes (with juice)	28 oz.	796 mL
Can of red kidney beans, rinsed and drained	19 oz.	540 mL
Frozen kernel corn	1 cup	250 mL
Pepper	1/4 tsp.	1 mL
Light sour cream	3 tbsp.	50 mL
Chopped fresh cilantro or parsley (optional)	3 tbsp.	50 mL

Heat first amount of cooking oil in large pot or Dutch oven on medium. Add sausage. Scramble-fry for about 5 minutes until browned. Transfer with slotted spoon to paper towels to drain. Discard drippings.

Heat second amount of cooking oil in same large pot. Add next 3 ingredients. Cook for 5 to 10 minutes, stirring often, until onion is softened.

Add chili powder and cumin. Heat and stir for about 1 minute until fragrant.

Add sausage and next 5 ingredients. Stir. Bring to a boil on medium-high. Reduce heat to medium-low. Cover. Simmer for about 15 minutes, stirring occasionally.

Add sour cream and cilantro. Stir. Serves 8.

1 serving: 221 Calories; 10.2 g Total Fat (4.8 g Mono, 1.6 g Poly, 3.2 g Sat); 16 mg Cholesterol; 23 g Carbohydrate; 5 g Fibre; 12 g Protein; 944 mg Sodium

Curried Lentil Vegetable Soup

Cool mint and yogurt topping adds a nice tangy freshness to this thick, mildly spiced soup.

MINTY YOGURT TOPPING

Low-fat plain yogurt	1/2 cup	125 mL
Chopped fresh mint leaves (or 1 1/2 tsp., 7 mL, dried)	2 tbsp.	30 mL
Cooking oil	1 tbsp.	15 mL
Finely chopped onion	1 1/2 cups	375 mL
Mild curry paste	2 tbsp.	30 mL
Low-sodium prepared chicken (or vegetable) broth	8 cups	2 L
Dried red split lentils	1 1/2 cups	375 mL
Cauliflower florets	4 cups	1 L
Frozen kernel corn	1 cup	250 mL
Frozen peas	1 cup	250 mL
Fresh spinach, stems removed, lightly packed	2 cups	500 mL

Minty Yogurt Topping: Combine yogurt and mint in small bowl. Chill. Makes about 1/2 cup (125 mL) topping.

Heat cooking oil in large pot or Dutch oven on medium. Add onion. Cook for 5 to 10 minutes, stirring often, until softened.

Add curry paste. Heat and stir for about 1 minute until fragrant.

Add broth and lentils. Stir. Bring to a boil on medium-high. Reduce heat to medium-low. Cover. Simmer for 15 minutes.

Add cauliflower. Stir. Cover. Simmer for about 10 minutes until cauliflower and lentils are tender.

Add corn and peas. Stir. Cover. Simmer for about 5 minutes until heated through.

Add spinach. Stir. Simmer, uncovered, for about 2 minutes until spinach is wilted. Garnish individual servings with topping. Serves 8.

1 serving: 248 Calories; 4.3 g Total Fat (1.9 g Mono, 1.2 g Poly, 0.5 g Sat); 1 mg Cholesterol; 38 g Carbohydrate; 7 g Fibre; 18 g Protein; 704 mg Sodium

Carrot and Orange Soup

A golden harvest soup, perfectly seasoned with thyme.

Cooking oil	1 tbsp.	15 mL
Finely chopped carrot	4 cups	1 L
Finely chopped onion	1 1/2 cups	375 mL
Prepared vegetable broth	5 cups	1.25 L
Dried thyme	1/2 tsp.	2 mL
Pepper	1/4 tsp.	1 mL
Orange juice	1/2 cup	125 mL
Light sour cream	1/4 cup	60 mL
Grated orange zest	1/2 tsp.	2 mL

Heat cooking oil in large pot or Dutch oven on medium-high. Add carrot and onion. Cook for 5 to 10 minutes, stirring often, until onion is softened.

Add next 3 ingredients. Stir. Cover. Bring to a boil. Boil gently for about 10 minutes, stirring occasionally, until carrot is tender.

Add remaining 3 ingredients. Stir. Remove from heat. Cool slightly. Carefully process with hand blender, or in blender in 2 batches, until smooth (see Safety Tip). Return to same large pot. Heat and stir on medium-high for 1 to 2 minutes until heated through. Serves 6.

1 serving: 104 Calories; 3.8 g Total Fat (2 g Mono, 0.9 g Poly, 1.3 g Sat); 2 mg Cholesterol; 14 g Carbohydrate; 3 g Fibre; 4 g Protein; 722 mg Sodium

Safety Tip: Follow blender manufacturer's instructions for processing hot liquids.

Paré Pointer

The chicken only went halfway across the road because she wanted to lay it on the line.

2 servings per portion

Tomato and Zucchini Soup

Caramelized onion adds a simple sweetness to this satisfying tomato soup. Great for lunch.

Olive (or cooking) oil	1 tbsp.	15 mL
Thinly sliced onion	2 cups	500 mL
Red wine vinegar	2 tsp.	10 mL
Granulated sugar	2 tsp.	10 mL
Pepper	1/4 tsp.	1 mL
Can of diced tomatoes (with juice)	28 oz.	796 mL
Low-sodium prepared chicken (or vegetable) broth	2 cups	500 mL
Medium zucchini (with peel), chopped	2	2
Frozen kernel corn	1 cup	250 mL
Chopped fresh basil	1/4 cup	60 mL

Heat olive oil in large saucepan on medium. Add onion. Cook for about 20 minutes, stirring often, until caramelized.

Add next 3 ingredients. Heat and stir for about 1 minute until sugar is dissolved.

Add next 4 ingredients. Stir. Bring to a boil on medium-high. Reduce heat to medium-low. Cover. Simmer for 5 to 10 minutes, stirring occasionally, until zucchini is tender.

Add basil. Stir. Serves 6.

1 serving: 112 Calories; 3 g Total Fat (1.8 g Mono, 0.5 g Poly, 0.4 g Sat); 0 mg Cholesterol; 20 g Carbohydrate; 3 g Fibre; 4 g Protein; 436 mg Sodium

Pictured on page 36.

Curried Sweet Potato Soup

Spicy curry and sweet potato make a nice blend. Serve with warm whole-wheat rolls.

Cooking oil	1 tbsp.	15 mL
Chopped onion	1 1/2 cups	375 mL
Curry powder	1 tbsp.	15 mL
Chopped fresh peeled orange-fleshed sweet potato	4 cups	1 L
Low-sodium prepared chicken broth	4 cups	1 L
Salt	1/4 tsp.	1 mL
Pepper	1/4 tsp.	1 mL
Low-fat plain yogurt	3 tbsp.	50 mL

Heat cooking oil in large pot or Dutch oven on medium. Add onion. Cook for about 20 minutes, stirring often, until caramelized.

Add curry powder. Heat and stir for about 1 minute until fragrant.

Add next 4 ingredients. Stir. Cover. Bring to a boil. Reduce heat to medium-low. Simmer for about 20 minutes, stirring occasionally, until sweet potato is tender. Remove from heat. Cool slightly. Carefully process with hand blender, or in blender in 2 batches, until smooth (see Safety Tip). Return to same large pot.

Add yogurt. Heat and stir on medium for about 2 minutes until heated through. Serves 4.

1 serving: 269 Calories; 4.2 g Total Fat (2.1 g Mono, 1.2 g Poly, 0.3 g Sat); 0 mg Cholesterol; 52 g Carbohydrate; 8 g Fibre; 7 g Protein; 812 mg Sodium

Safety Tip: Follow blender manufacturer's instructions for processing hot liquids.

Minted Beef and Noodles

Curried beef skewers nestle on a bed of rice noodles and colourful veggies.
Exotic flavours make this perfect for a summer meal on the patio.

SWEET AND SPICY MARINADE

Sweet chili sauce	1 tbsp.	15 mL
Fish sauce	1 tbsp.	15 mL
Curry paste	2 tsp.	10 mL
Finely grated ginger root	1 tsp.	5 mL
Garlic cloves, minced (or 1/2 tsp., 2 mL, powder)	2	2
Beef top sirloin steak, cut lengthwise into 1/4 inch (6 mm) slices	1 lb.	454 g
Bamboo skewers (8 inches, 20 cm, each), soaked in water for 10 minutes	8	8
Rice vermicelli	4 oz.	113 g
Boiling water		
English cucumber (with peel), halved lengthwise, seeds removed, thinly sliced	1	1
Julienned carrot (see Note)	1 cup	250 mL
Fresh bean sprouts	1 cup	250 mL
Chopped fresh mint leaves (or 3/4 tsp., 4 mL, dried)	1 tbsp.	15 mL

SPICY LIME DRESSING

Lime juice	1/4 cup	60 mL
Sweet chili sauce	2 tbsp.	30 mL
Curry paste	4 tsp.	20 mL
Peanut (or cooking) oil	2 tsp.	10 mL
Coarsely chopped unsalted peanuts, toasted (see Tip, page 47)	2 tbsp.	30 mL

Sweet and Spicy Marinade: Combine first 5 ingredients in small cup. Makes about 2 tbsp. (30 mL) marinade.

Put beef into large resealable freezer bag. Pour marinade over top. Seal bag. Turn until coated. Marinate in refrigerator for at least 6 hours or overnight, turning occasionally.

Preheat electric grill for 5 minutes or gas barbecue to medium (see Note). Thread beef slices, accordion-style, onto skewers. Cook on greased grill for 3 to 4 minutes per side until desired doneness. Transfer to large plate. Cover to keep warm.

(continued on next page)

Put vermicelli into large bowl. Pour boiling water over top until covered. Let stand for about 5 minutes until vermicelli is tender. Drain. Rinse with cold water. Drain well. Return to same large bowl.

Add next 4 ingredients. Toss.

Spicy Lime Dressing: Combine first 4 ingredients in jar with tight-fitting lid. Shake well. Makes about 1/4 cup (60 mL) dressing. Drizzle over vermicelli mixture. Toss well. Remove to large serving dish. Arrange beef skewers over top.

Sprinkle with peanuts. Serves 4.

1 serving: 531 Calories; 17.4 g Total Fat (7.5 g Mono, 2.4 g Poly, 4.9 g Sat); 56 mg Cholesterol; 65 g Carbohydrate; 4 g Fibre; 29 g Protein; 517 mg Sodium

Pictured on front cover and page 89.

Note: To julienne vegetables, cut into 1/8 inch (3 mm) strips that resemble matchsticks.

Note: Skewers may be broiled in oven. Place on greased broiler pan. Broil about 4 inches (10 cm) from heat in oven for 3 to 4 minutes per side until desired doneness.

MINTED CHICKEN AND NOODLES: Omit beef. Use same amount of boneless, skinless chicken breast halves, cut into 1/4 inch (6 mm) slices.

 To toast nuts, seeds or coconut, spread evenly in ungreased shallow pan. Bake in 350°F (175°C) oven for 5 to 10 minutes, stirring or shaking often, until desired doneness.

Beef Pot Roast

Oh-so-tender roast in a rich, wine-flavoured "jus." A warming meal.

Boneless beef blade (or chuck) roast	2 lbs.	900 g
Garlic cloves, quartered lengthwise	4	4
Italian seasoning	1 tsp.	5 mL
Pepper, sprinkle		
Cooking oil	1 tbsp.	15 mL
Chopped carrot	2 cups	500 mL
Chopped parsnip	2 cups	500 mL
Chopped onion	2 cups	500 mL
Low-sodium prepared beef broth	1 1/4 cups	300 mL
Chopped yellow turnip (rutabaga)	1 cup	250 mL
Dry (or alcohol-free) red wine	1/2 cup	125 mL

Cut 16 shallow slits in roast at random. Insert 1 piece of garlic into each slit. Sprinkle roast with Italian seasoning and pepper.

Heat cooking oil in large pot or Dutch oven on medium-high. Add roast. Cook for about 5 minutes, turning occasionally, until browned on all sides. Transfer to large plate.

Combine remaining 6 ingredients in same large pot. Return roast to pot. Bring to a boil on medium. Reduce heat to medium-low. Cover. Simmer for 1 3/4 to 2 hours, turning roast at halftime, until tender. Remove roast to large plate. Cover to keep warm. Remove vegetables with slotted spoon to large serving bowl. Cover to keep warm. Bring liquid in pot to a boil on medium-high. Boil, uncovered, for 10 to 15 minutes until reduced by about half. Remove to small serving bowl. Cut roast into thin slices. Serve with vegetables and "jus." Serves 8 (2 to 3 oz., 57 to 85 g, roast beef per serving).

1 serving: 334 Calories; 18.7 g Total Fat (8.4 g Mono, 1.2 g Poly, 6.9 g Sat); 66 mg Cholesterol; 17 g Carbohydrate; 3 g Fibre; 22 g Protein; 275 mg Sodium

 Keep a daily food diary to track what you eat and when. This journal will help identify things to improve upon once you compare it to *Canada's Food Guide.*

Ginger Pear Pork

Tender chunks of pear and a well-seasoned sauce dress up pork for dinner.
Serve with brown rice.

Pork tenderloin, trimmed of fat	1 lb.	454 g
Pepper	1/4 tsp.	1 mL
Olive (or cooking) oil	1 tbsp.	15 mL
Chopped onion	2 tbsp.	30 mL
Finely grated ginger root	1 tbsp.	15 mL
Fresh peeled medium pears, diced	2	2
Apple cider	1 cup	250 mL
Lime juice	1 tbsp.	15 mL
Liquid honey	1 tsp.	5 mL
Chopped fresh thyme leaves (or 1/4 tsp., 1 mL, dried)	1 tsp.	5 mL

Sprinkle tenderloin with pepper. Heat olive oil in medium frying pan on medium-high. Add tenderloin. Cook for about 5 minutes, turning occasionally, until browned on all sides. Reduce heat to medium. Cover. Cook for 10 to 12 minutes until meat thermometer inserted into thickest part of tenderloin reads 155°F (68°C). Remove to large plate. Cover with foil. Let stand for 10 minutes. Internal temperature should rise to at least 160°F (70°C).

Heat and stir onion and ginger in same medium frying pan for about 1 minute until onion is softened.

Add pear. Cook for 1 to 2 minutes, stirring occasionally, until pear starts to soften.

Add remaining 4 ingredients. Bring to a boil. Boil gently, uncovered, for about 8 minutes until pear is softened and liquid is almost evaporated. Transfer to small serving bowl. Cut tenderloin crosswise into 1/2 inch (12 mm) slices. Serve with sauce. Makes 4 servings (2 to 3 oz., 57 to 85 g, pork per serving).

1 serving: 254 Calories; 8.4 g Total Fat (4.7 g Mono, 0.8 g Poly, 2.1 g Sat); 72 mg Cholesterol; 20 g Carbohydrate; 3 g Fibre; 24 g Protein; 63 mg Sodium

Wine and Rosemary Chicken

Tender chicken in a subtle white wine and rosemary sauce. Garnish with a sprig of rosemary for a pretty presentation.

Cooking oil	2 tsp.	10 mL
Boneless, skinless chicken thighs, halved	1 lb.	454 g
Baby carrots	1 1/2 cups	375 mL
Chopped onion	1 cup	250 mL
Dry (or alcohol-free) white wine	1 cup	250 mL
Low-sodium prepared chicken broth	1/2 cup	125 mL
Fresh rosemary sprigs	2	2
Garlic cloves, minced	2	2
(or 1/2 tsp., 2 mL, powder)		
Lemon pepper	1/2 tsp.	2 mL
Water	1 tbsp.	15 mL
Cornstarch	2 tsp.	10 mL
Light sour cream	2 tbsp.	30 mL

Heat cooking oil in large pot or Dutch oven on medium-high. Add chicken. Cook for about 10 minutes, stirring occasionally, until browned.

Add next 7 ingredients. Stir. Bring to a boil. Reduce heat to medium-low. Cover. Simmer for about 40 minutes, stirring occasionally, until chicken and carrots are tender.

Stir water into cornstarch in small cup until smooth. Add to chicken mixture. Heat and stir on medium for about 1 minute until sauce is boiling and thickened. Discard rosemary sprigs.

Add sour cream. Stir well. Serves 4.

1 serving: *285 Calories; 9.7 g Total Fat (3.7 g Mono, 2.5 g Poly, 2.6 g Sat); 104 mg Cholesterol; 13 g Carbohydrate; 2 g Fibre; 26 g Protein; 206 mg Sodium*

 Low-fat and non-fat dairy products have less fat and calories but still provide the protein and calcium essential to healthy eating. Be sure to read the labels and choose products with a lower percent M.F. (milk fat) or B.F. (butter fat).

Braised Lamb Chops

A splash of wine and a little thyme are all it takes to make a full-bodied "jus"
for moist, tender lamb and tender-crisp vegetables. Serve with oven-roasted potatoes
for a complete meal.

All-purpose flour	3 tbsp.	50 mL
Cajun seasoning	1 1/2 tbsp.	25 mL
Lamb loin chops (about 2 lbs., 900 g)	8	8
Cooking oil	1 tbsp.	15 mL
Baby carrots	2 cups	500 mL
Low-sodium prepared chicken broth	1 cup	250 mL
Dry (or alcohol-free) white wine	1/2 cup	125 mL
Medium onions, cut into thin wedges	2	2
Chopped fresh thyme leaves	1 tbsp.	15 mL
(or 3/4 tsp., 4 mL, dried)		
Greek seasoning	1/2 tsp.	2 mL
Bay leaves	2	2
Pepper	1/4 tsp.	1 mL
Frozen cut green beans	1 cup	250 mL

Combine flour and Cajun seasoning in large shallow dish. Press both sides of each lamb chop into flour mixture until coated.

Heat cooking oil in large pot or Dutch oven on medium-high. Add chops. Cook for 2 to 3 minutes per side until browned.

Add next 8 ingredients. Stir. Bring to a boil. Reduce heat to medium-low. Cover. Simmer for about 1 1/4 hours, stirring occasionally, until chops are tender. Remove cover. Bring to a boil on medium. Boil gently for about 15 minutes until sauce is thickened. Discard bay leaves.

Add green beans. Stir. Cover. Cook for 3 to 5 minutes until green beans are tender-crisp. Serves 8.

1 serving: 372 Calories; 27.4 g Total Fat (11.4 g Mono, 2.6 g Poly, 11.3 g Sat); 70 mg Cholesterol; 11 g Carbohydrate; 2 g Fibre; 17 g Protein; 393 mg Sodium

Artichoke Tomato Chicken

Chicken never tasted so good. Enjoy this light, summery dish with a salad on the side.

Boneless, skinless chicken breast halves (4 – 6 oz., 113 – 170 g, each)	4	4
Garlic and herb no-salt seasoning (such as Mrs. Dash), sprinkle		
Pepper, sprinkle		
Cooking oil	1 tbsp.	15 mL
Can of artichoke hearts, drained and quartered	14 oz.	398 mL
Roma (plum) tomatoes, thickly sliced lengthwise	4	4
Chopped fresh oregano leaves	1 tbsp.	15 mL
Balsamic vinegar	1 tsp.	5 mL
Granulated sugar	1 tsp.	5 mL
Garlic and herb no-salt seasoning (such as Mrs. Dash), sprinkle		

Sprinkle both sides of each chicken breast half with first amount of no-salt seasoning and pepper.

Heat cooking oil in large frying pan on medium-high. Add chicken. Cook for 3 to 4 minutes per side until browned. Arrange in single layer in greased 1 1/2 quart (1.5 L) shallow baking dish.

Layer artichoke evenly on top of chicken. Layer tomato slices evenly on top of artichoke.

Sprinkle remaining 4 ingredients over top. Bake, uncovered, in 350°F (175°C) oven for about 30 minutes until chicken is no longer pink inside. Serves 4.

1 serving: *269 Calories; 6.7 g Total Fat (2.7 g Mono, 1.9 g Poly, 1 g Sat); 81 mg Cholesterol; 19 g Carbohydrate; 5 g Fibre; 35 g Protein; 198 mg Sodium*

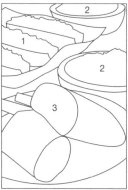

1. Crab-Stuffed Zucchini, page 64
2. Bean, Ham and Potato Salad, page 20
3. Turkey Wraps, page 59

Props courtesy of: Pier 1 Imports
　　　　　　　　　　Cherison Enterprises Inc.

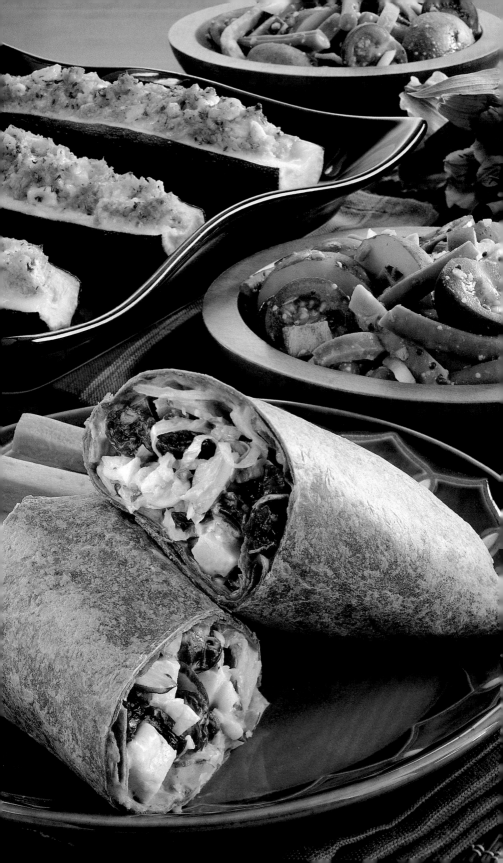

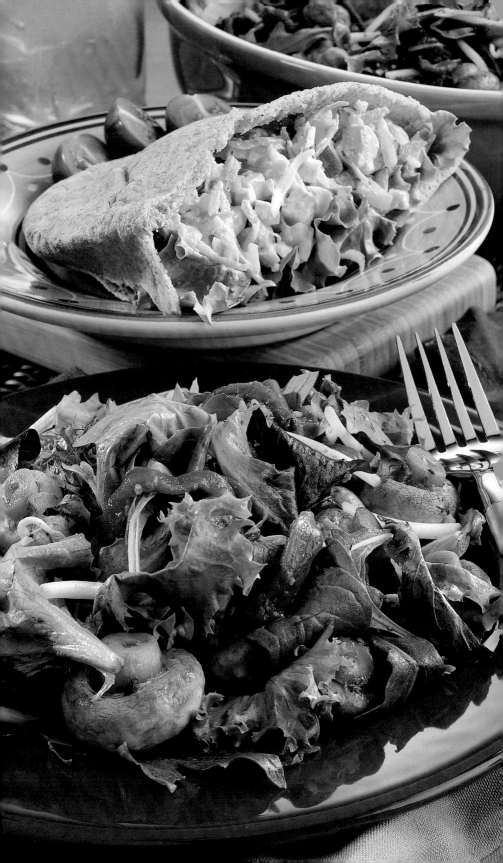

Pumpkin Enchiladas

A subtle bite of chili in a pumpkin-packed tortilla. A tasty autumn dinner.

Cooked long-grain white rice (about 1/2 cup, 125 mL, uncooked)	1 1/2 cups	375 mL
Thinly sliced green onion	1 cup	250 mL
Frozen peas	1 cup	250 mL
Grated Monterey Jack cheese	1/2 cup	125 mL
Flour tortillas (9 inch, 22 cm, diameter)	6	6
PUMPKIN SAUCE		
Can of pure pumpkin (no spices)	14 oz.	398 mL
Water	1 1/2 cups	375 mL
Chili powder	2 tsp.	10 mL
Grated Monterey Jack cheese	1 cup	250 mL

Combine first 4 ingredients in large bowl. Spoon across centre of each tortilla. Fold sides over filling. Roll up from bottom to enclose. Arrange in single layer in greased 3 quart (3 L) shallow baking dish.

Pumpkin Sauce: Combine first 3 ingredients in medium bowl. Makes about 3 cups (750 mL) sauce. Spread evenly over enchiladas.

Sprinkle with cheese. Bake in 450°F (230°C) oven for about 15 minutes until heated through. Broil 6 inches (15 cm) from heat for about 5 minutes until cheese is melted and golden. Serves 6.

1 serving: 370 Calories; 12.6 g Total Fat (3.9 g Mono, 1.6 g Poly, 6.3 g Sat); 27 mg Cholesterol; 50 g Carbohydrate; 5 g Fibre; 15 g Protein; 405 mg Sodium

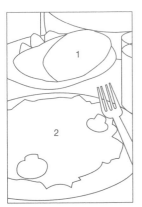

1. Crunchy Chicken Pitas, page 58
2. Warm Mushroom Salad, page 26

Props courtesy of: Pier 1 Imports
   Danesco Inc.
   Cherison Enterprises Inc.
   Totally Bamboo

Ruby Chard Pork

Earthy ruby chard and pleasantly sweet fruit complement tender pork medallions in this colourful dish.

Olive (or cooking) oil	1 tbsp.	15 mL
Pork tenderloin, trimmed of fat and cut into 1/2 inch (12 mm) medallions	1 lb.	454 g
Lemon juice	2 tbsp.	30 mL
Garlic cloves, minced (or 1/2 tsp., 2 mL, powder)	2	2
Ruby chard, coarsely chopped, lightly packed	2 lbs.	900 g
Currants	1/2 cup	125 mL
Chopped dried apricot	1/3 cup	75 mL
Pepper	1/8 tsp.	0.5 mL
Orange juice	2 tbsp.	30 mL
Cornstarch	2 tsp.	10 mL
Pine nuts, toasted (see Tip, page 47)	1/4 cup	60 mL

Heat olive oil in large pot or Dutch oven on medium-high. Add pork medallions. Cook for about 2 minutes per side until browned. Transfer to large plate. Cover to keep warm.

Combine lemon juice and garlic in same large pot. Heat and stir on medium for about 1 minute until fragrant.

Add next 4 ingredients. Cover. Cook for about 5 minutes until chard starts to wilt. Stir carefully. Cover. Cook for another 5 minutes until stalks are tender-crisp.

Stir orange juice into cornstarch in small cup until smooth. Add to chard mixture. Add pork medallions. Heat and stir until sauce is boiling and thickened. Remove to large serving dish.

Sprinkle with pine nuts. Serves 4.

1 serving: 321 Calories; 13.9 g Total Fat (6.7 g Mono, 3 g Poly, 2.9 g Sat); 72 mg Cholesterol; 23 g Carbohydrate; 6 g Fibre; 31 g Protein; 540 mg Sodium

Spiced Salmon and Salsa

Cool as a cucumber, the salsa tames the heat of deliciously spicy salmon.

Cajun seasoning	1 tbsp.	15 mL
Lemon pepper	2 tsp.	10 mL
Salmon fillets, skin and any small bones removed	4	4

MELON CUCUMBER SALSA

Diced cantaloupe	3/4 cup	175 mL
Diced honeydew	3/4 cup	175 mL
English cucumber (with peel), quartered lengthwise, seeds removed, diced	1/4	1/4
Finely chopped red onion	1/3 cup	75 mL
Lime juice	3 tbsp.	50 mL
Chopped fresh cilantro or parsley (or 1 1/2 tsp., 7 mL, dried)	2 tbsp.	30 mL
Hot pepper sauce	1/2 tsp.	2 mL
Pepper, sprinkle		

Combine Cajun seasoning and lemon pepper in small bowl. Rub on both sides of each fillet. Let stand for 15 minutes. Preheat electric grill for 5 minutes or gas barbecue to medium-high (see Note). Cook fillets on greased grill for 3 to 4 minutes per side until fish flakes easily when tested with fork.

Melon Cucumber Salsa: Combine all 8 ingredients in medium bowl. Makes about 2 cups (500 mL) salsa. Serve with salmon. Serves 4.

1 serving: 587 Calories; 24.8 g Total Fat (8.1 g Mono, 9.8 g Poly, 3.8 g Sat); 211 mg Cholesterol; 10 g Carbohydrate; 1 g Fibre; 77 g Protein; 800 mg Sodium

Note: Salmon may be broiled in oven. Place on greased broiler pan. Broil about 4 inches (10 cm) from heat for 3 to 4 minutes per side until fish flakes easily when tested with fork.

tip To reduce fat, bake, broil, roast, grill or microwave food instead of frying. Or use a non-stick frying pan with little or no oil, and drain off excess fat after frying.

Crunchy Chicken Pitas

Creamy, crunchy filling stuffed into a whole-wheat pita. A delicious light lunch.

CRUNCHY CHICKEN FILLING

Grated carrot	3/4 cup	175 mL
Finely chopped cooked chicken	3/4 cup	175 mL
Finely chopped celery	1/2 cup	125 mL
Chopped dill pickle	6 tbsp.	100 mL
Grated light sharp Cheddar cheese	1/3 cup	75 mL
Light mayonnaise	1/4 cup	60 mL
Sliced almonds, toasted (see Tip, page 47)	2 tbsp.	30 mL
Pepper, sprinkle		
Whole-wheat pita bread (7 inch, 18 cm, diameter), halved	1	1
Lettuce leaves	2	2

Crunchy Chicken Filling: Combine first 8 ingredients in medium bowl.

Line each pita bread half with 1 lettuce leaf. Spoon filling into each pocket. Makes 2 chicken pitas.

1 chicken pita: 388 Calories; 18.9 g Total Fat (9.4 g Mono, 4.3 g Poly, 4 g Sat); 60 mg Cholesterol; 29 g Carbohydrate; 5 g Fibre; 27 g Protein; 883 mg Sodium

Pictured on page 54.

Paré Pointer

It isn't hard to meet expenses—they're around every corner.

Turkey Wraps

Turkey salad with a cranberry twist—all wrapped up for lunch.

Whole cranberry sauce	1/4 cup	60 mL
Light sour cream	1/4 cup	60 mL
Light mayonnaise	1/4 cup	60 mL
Whole-wheat flour tortillas	4	4
(9 inch, 22 cm, diameter)		
Finely shredded iceberg lettuce,	1 cup	250 mL
lightly packed		
Chopped cooked turkey	1 1/4 cups	300 mL
Finely chopped celery	1/2 cup	125 mL
Finely chopped green onion	1/2 cup	125 mL
Raisins	1/2 cup	125 mL
Sliced almonds, toasted	1/4 cup	60 mL
(see Tip, page 47)		

Combine first 3 ingredients in large bowl. Spread 1 1/2 tbsp. (25 mL) on each tortilla, leaving 1 inch (2.5 cm) edge.

Add remaining 6 ingredients to remaining cranberry mixture. Mix well. Spoon across centre of each tortilla. Fold sides over filling. Roll up from bottom to enclose. Makes 4 wraps.

1 wrap: 428 Calories; 13.4 g Total Fat (6.4 g Mono, 3.6 g Poly, 3 g Sat); 39 mg Cholesterol; 59 g Carbohydrate; 7 g Fibre; 22 g Protein; 472 mg Sodium

Pictured on page 53.

Grilled Veggie Burgers

Mildly spiced mayonnaise adds zip to layers of grilled veggies nestled in whole-grain buns.

Medium red pepper, quartered	1	1
Fresh peeled medium orange-fleshed sweet potato, cut into 1/8 inch (3 mm) slices	1	1
Medium zucchini (with peel), cut lengthwise into 1/4 inch (6 mm) slices	1	1
Cooking oil	1 tsp.	5 mL
Thinly sliced onion	1 cup	250 mL
Sweet chili sauce	2 tsp.	10 mL
Lime juice	2 tsp.	10 mL
CHILI LIME MAYONNAISE		
Light mayonnaise	1/4 cup	60 mL
Sweet chili sauce	2 tbsp.	30 mL
Lime juice	1 tbsp.	15 mL
Whole-grain buns, split, toasted	4	4
Fresh spinach, stems removed, lightly packed	1 cup	250 mL

Preheat electric grill for 5 minutes or gas barbecue to medium-high. Cook red pepper, skin-side up, on greased grill for about 10 minutes until tender-crisp. Transfer to small bowl. Cover to keep warm.

Spray both sides of each sweet potato slice with cooking spray. Cook on greased grill for about 3 minutes per side until tender. Transfer to large plate. Cover to keep warm.

Spray both sides of each zucchini slice with cooking spray. Cook on greased grill for about 2 minutes per side until tender and grill marks appear. Transfer to separate large plate. Cut zucchini slices in half crosswise. Cover to keep warm.

Heat cooking oil in large frying pan on medium. Add onion. Cook for 5 to 10 minutes, stirring often, until softened.

Add first amounts of chili sauce and lime juice. Stir. Remove from heat. Cover to keep warm.

Chili Lime Mayonnaise: Combine first 3 ingredients in small bowl. Makes about 1/3 cup (75 mL) mayonnaise. Spread on both halves of each bun.

(continued on next page)

Layer onion mixture, sweet potato, red pepper, zucchini and spinach on bottom half of each bun. Cover with top halves. Makes 4 veggie burgers.

1 veggie burger: 216 Calories; 7.4 g Total Fat (3.8 g Mono, 2.5 g Poly, 0.7 g Sat); 0 mg Cholesterol; 35 g Carbohydrate; 4 g Fibre; 5 g Protein; 408 mg Sodium

GRILLED VEGGIE BURRITOS: Omit buns. Spread Chili Lime Mayonnaise on each of 4 whole wheat flour tortillas, almost to edge. Layer prepared ingredients across centre of each tortilla. Fold sides over filling. Roll up from bottom to enclose. Makes 4 veggie burritos.

Mediterranean Sub

A sea of rich Mediterranean flavour awaits in this satisfying sandwich.

Hummus	3 tbsp.	50 mL
Section of baguette (8 inch, 20 cm, length), split	1	1
Fresh spinach (or arugula), stems removed, lightly packed	3/4 cup	175 mL
Roasted red peppers, drained, blotted dry, cut into thin strips	1/3 cup	75 mL
Thinly sliced red onion, separated into rings	1/4 cup	60 mL
Ripe medium olives, thinly sliced	4	4
Low-fat deli ham slices	2	2
Pepper, sprinkle		

Spread hummus on both baguette halves.

Layer next 5 ingredients, in order given, on bottom half.

Sprinkle with pepper. Cover with top half. Cut in half. Makes 2 sandwiches.

1 sandwich: 470 Calories; 10.6 g Total Fat (5.4 g Mono, 2.1 g Poly, 2.1 g Sat); 18 mg Cholesterol; 72 g Carbohydrate; 5 g Fibre; 22 g Protein; 1413 mg Sodium

Pictured on page 36.

Potato Cakes Benny

Poached eggs top cheesy mushroom potato patties. An all-in-one breakfast or light lunch!

Hard margarine (or butter)	1 tbsp.	15 mL
Chopped fresh white mushrooms	1 cup	250 mL
Garlic clove, minced	1	1
(or 1/4 tsp., 1 mL, powder)		
Mashed potatoes (about 3 medium,	2 cups	500 mL
uncooked)		
Large egg, fork-beaten	1	1
Chopped fresh chives	2 tsp.	10 mL
(or 1/2 tsp., 2 mL, dried)		
Pepper	1/4 tsp.	1 mL
All-purpose flour	1/4 cup	60 mL
Paprika	1/4 tsp.	1 mL
Cooking oil	2 tsp.	10 mL
Grated medium Cheddar cheese	1 cup	250 mL
Water		
White vinegar	1 tsp.	5 mL
Large eggs	8	8

Melt margarine in small frying pan on medium-high. Add mushrooms and garlic. Cook for 2 to 3 minutes, stirring often, until mushrooms are softened. Transfer to medium bowl.

Add next 4 ingredients. Stir well. Shape mixture into 8 patties, using about 1/4 cup (60 mL) for each.

Combine flour and paprika in small shallow dish. Press both sides of each patty into flour mixture until coated.

Heat cooking oil in large frying pan on medium-high. Add patties. Cook for 1 to 2 minutes per side until golden. Transfer to baking sheet.

Sprinkle cheese over each patty. Cover to keep warm.

Pour water into large saucepan until 3 inches (7.5 cm) deep. Add vinegar. Stir. Bring to a boil on medium. Reduce heat to medium-low. Water should continue to simmer.

(continued on next page)

Break eggs, 1 at a time, into shallow dish. Slip each egg into water until all eggs are submerged (see Note). Cook each egg for 2 to 3 minutes until white is set and yolk reaches desired doneness. Remove each cooked egg with slotted spoon. Place 1 egg on top of each patty. Transfer 2 egg-topped potato cakes to each of 4 plates. Serves 4.

1 serving: 477 Calories; 26.7 g Total Fat (10.4 g Mono, 2.9 g Poly, 10.6 g Sat); 516 mg Cholesterol; 34 g Carbohydrate; 2 g Fibre; 25 g Protein; 368 mg Sodium

Note: Use a stove-top egg poacher, if desired.

Pictured on page 71.

Grilled Veggie Quesadillas

Something for everyone! Adults will enjoy the colourful vegetables. Kids will like the gooey cheese. Serve with salsa and sour cream.

Fat-free Italian dressing	2 tbsp.	30 mL
Mild pickled banana peppers, finely chopped (optional)	1 tbsp.	15 mL
Olive (or cooking) oil	1 tsp.	5 mL
Garlic clove, minced (or 1/4 tsp., 1 mL, powder)	1	1
Medium zucchini, quartered lengthwise	1	1
Small red pepper, quartered	1	1
Whole-wheat flour tortillas (9 inch, 22 cm, diameter)	4	4
Grated sharp Cheddar cheese	2 cups	500 mL
Green onions, sliced	2	2

Combine first 4 ingredients in medium bowl.

Add zucchini and red pepper. Stir until coated. Preheat two-sided grill for 5 minutes. Place vegetables in single layer on greased grill. Close lid. Cook for about 7 minutes until tender-crisp and lightly browned. Dice vegetables.

Scatter vegetables, cheese and green onions over half of each tortilla. Fold other half over filling. Press down lightly. Cook tortillas, 1 or 2 at a time, on greased grill for 3 to 4 minutes until grill marks appear. Cut each quesadilla into 3 wedges. Serves 4.

1 serving: 440 Calories; 22.7 g Total Fat (6.7 g Mono, 1.4 g Poly, 13 g Sat); 63 mg Cholesterol; 40 g Carbohydrate; 6 g Fibre; 22 g Protein; 798 mg Sodium

Crab-Stuffed Zucchini

What to do with a bountiful zucchini harvest? Stuff it with an elegant crab filling.
Garlic and dill add the perfect accents.

Medium zucchini, halved lengthwise	3	3
Hard margarine (or butter)	2 tbsp.	30 mL
Finely chopped onion	1/2 cup	125 mL
Garlic cloves, minced (or 1/2 tsp., 2 mL, powder)	2	2
Can of crabmeat, drained, cartilage removed, flaked	6 oz.	170 g
Grated Swiss cheese	1/2 cup	125 mL
Crumbled feta cheese	1/3 cup	75 mL
Large egg, fork-beaten	1	1
All-purpose flour	1 tbsp.	15 mL
Chopped fresh parsley (or 3/4 tsp., 4 mL, flakes)	1 tbsp.	15 mL
Chopped fresh dill (or 1/2 tsp., 2 mL, dried)	2 tsp.	10 mL
Paprika	1 tsp.	5 mL
Pepper	1/4 tsp.	1 mL

Scoop out pulp from each zucchini half, leaving 1/2 inch (12 mm) thick shells.
Arrange shells in single layer on greased baking sheet. Chop pulp.

Melt margarine in small frying pan on medium-high. Add onion and garlic. Cook
for 3 to 5 minutes, stirring often, until onion starts to soften. Add zucchini pulp.
Stir. Transfer to medium bowl.

Add remaining 9 ingredients. Stir well. Spoon into zucchini shells. Bake in 375°F
(190°C) oven for about 30 minutes until filling is set. Makes 6 stuffed zucchini.

*1 stuffed zucchini: 150 Calories; 9.7 g Total Fat (4 g Mono, 0.7 g Poly, 4.1 g Sat);
53 mg Cholesterol; 6 g Carbohydrate; 2 g Fibre; 10 g Protein; 369 mg Sodium*

Pictured on page 53.

Fruit-Full French Toast

Your efforts will be fruitful as raves are sure to come your way when you make this delightful dish.

Orange marmalade	1/4 cup	60 mL
Thick whole-wheat bread slices	6	6
Chopped dried apricot	1/2 cup	125 mL
Dried cranberries	1/4 cup	60 mL
Large eggs	4	4
Milk	3/4 cup	175 mL
Applesauce	1/2 cup	125 mL
Vanilla	1/2 tsp.	2 mL
Ground cinnamon	1/2 tsp.	2 mL
Fresh raspberries	1 cup	250 mL
Fresh blueberries	1/2 cup	125 mL
Sliced natural almonds, toasted (see Tip, page 47), optional	2 tbsp.	30 mL
Icing (confectioner's) sugar (optional)	1 tsp.	5 mL

Spread marmalade on 1 side of each bread slice. Cut slices in half diagonally.

Scatter apricot and cranberries in greased 9 x 13 inch (22 x 33 cm) pan. Arrange bread slices, marmalade-side up, in single layer on top of fruit.

Beat eggs and milk with whisk in medium bowl.

Add applesauce, vanilla and cinnamon. Stir well. Carefully pour over bread. Cover. Chill overnight. Bake, uncovered, in 450°F (230°C) oven for 20 to 25 minutes until edges are golden.

Scatter raspberries, blueberries and almonds, in order given, over top.

Sprinkle with icing sugar. Serves 6.

1 serving: 302 Calories; 6.3 g Total Fat (2.4 g Mono, 1.1 g Poly, 1.8 g Sat); 145 mg Cholesterol; 54 g Carbohydrate; 7 g Fibre; 12 g Protein; 368 mg Sodium

Pictured on page 71.

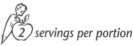
servings per portion

Ratatouille Pie

Traditional ratatouille wrapped with rice in a phyllo crust. Impressive!

Diced eggplant	3 cups	750 mL
Diced zucchini (with peel)	3 cups	750 mL
Salt	1 tbsp.	15 mL
Cooking oil	1 tbsp.	15 mL
Chopped onion	1 cup	250 mL
Garlic cloves, minced	2	2
(or 1/2 tsp., 2 mL, powder)		
Dried thyme	1/2 tsp.	2 mL
Dried basil	1/2 tsp.	2 mL
Dried oregano	1/4 tsp.	1 mL
Pepper	1/4 tsp.	1 mL
Can of diced tomatoes, drained	14 oz.	398 mL
Diced green pepper	1 cup	250 mL
Phyllo pastry sheets, thawed	10	10
according to package directions		
Cooked long-grain white rice	3 cups	750 mL
(about 1 cup, 250 mL, uncooked)		
Hard margarine (or butter), melted	1 tbsp.	15 mL

Put eggplant and zucchini into large bowl. Sprinkle with salt. Stir. Let stand for 1 hour. Drain. Rinse with cold water. Drain. Gently squeeze to remove excess liquid. Set aside.

Heat cooking oil in large frying pan on medium. Add next 6 ingredients. Cook for about 5 minutes, stirring often, until onion starts to soften.

Add eggplant mixture, tomatoes and green pepper. Stir. Cook for about 5 minutes, stirring occasionally, until green pepper is tender-crisp. Mixture will be quite dry. Cool.

Work with pastry sheets 1 at a time. Keep remaining sheets covered with damp tea towel to prevent drying. Spray 1 side of sheet with cooking spray. Fold into thirds lengthwise to make 4 inch (10 cm) strip. Place in greased 9 inch (22 cm) springform pan, allowing strip to hang over edge. Spray second pastry sheet with cooking spray. Fold into thirds lengthwise. Lay over first pastry strip at an angle, slightly overlapping. Repeat with 3 more pastry sheets and cooking spray until entire pan is covered (see Diagram 1). Gently press pastry to fit in pan, forming shell.

(continued on next page)

Press half of rice firmly in bottom of pastry shell. Spread half of vegetable mixture evenly over rice (see Diagram 2). Fold remaining pastry sheets. Cover filling, overlapping at an angle. Layer remaining rice and vegetable mixture over pastry. Fold overhanging pastry over filling toward centre of pie. Filling will not be completely covered.

Brush pastry with margarine. Bake in 350°F (175°C) oven for about 1 hour until pastry is crisp and golden. Let stand for 15 minutes. Cuts into 8 wedges.

1 wedge: 246 Calories; 5.2 g Total Fat (2.4 g Mono, 1.7 g Poly, 0.8 g Sat); 0 mg Cholesterol; 45 g Carbohydrate; 3 g Fibre; 6 g Protein; 1102 mg Sodium

Pictured on page 72.

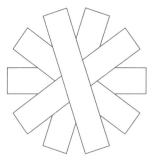

Diagram 1

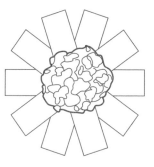

Diagram 2

Paré Pointer

One of Jimmy's bicycle wheels said to the other,
"Was it you who spoke?"

Calico Rice Creole

Vegetables and rice in a spicy tomato sauce—this will remind you of jambalaya, without the meat! Add more cayenne pepper if you like lots of heat.

Cooking oil	1 tbsp.	15 mL
Chopped red onion	2 cups	500 mL
Garlic cloves, minced (or 1 tsp., 5 mL, powder)	4	4
Cajun seasoning	1 tbsp.	15 mL
Ground cumin	1 tsp.	5 mL
Cayenne pepper	1/8 tsp.	0.5 mL
Can of diced tomatoes (with juice)	28 oz.	796 mL
Can of mixed beans, rinsed and drained	19 oz.	540 mL
Prepared vegetable broth	2 cups	500 mL
Frozen kernel corn	2 cups	500 mL
Chopped red pepper	2 cups	500 mL
Chopped celery	1 cup	250 mL
Chopped carrot	1 cup	250 mL
Worcestershire sauce	1 tbsp.	15 mL
Long-grain white rice	1/2 cup	125 mL
Chopped fresh (or frozen, thawed) green beans	1 1/2 cups	375 mL
Chopped fresh parsley (or 1 1/2 tsp., 7 mL, flakes)	2 tbsp.	30 mL

Heat cooking oil in large pot or Dutch oven on medium. Add onion. Cook for 5 to 10 minutes, stirring often, until softened.

Add next 4 ingredients. Heat and stir for about 1 minute until fragrant.

Add next 8 ingredients. Stir. Bring to a boil on high. Reduce heat to medium-low. Cover. Simmer for 30 minutes, stirring occasionally.

Add rice. Stir. Cover. Simmer for about 20 minutes, without stirring, until rice is almost tender.

Add green beans. Stir. Cover. Simmer for about 7 minutes until green beans are tender-crisp.

Add parsley. Stir gently. Serves 6.

1 serving: 292 Calories; 4.4 g Total Fat (1.8 g Mono, 1.4 g Poly, 0.5 g Sat); 0 mg Cholesterol; 57 g Carbohydrate; 8 g Fibre; 11 g Protein; 877 mg Sodium

Pictured on page 72.

Sweet Potato Pork Tenders

Sweet apple, spicy cinnamon and a nutty topping. If it weren't for the pork, your family could mistake this for dessert!

All-purpose flour	1 tbsp.	15 mL
Cornstarch	1 tbsp.	15 mL
Garlic salt	1/4 tsp.	1 mL
Pepper	1/8 tsp.	0.5 mL
Pork tenderloin, trimmed of fat and cut into 3/4 inch (2 cm) pieces	1 lb.	454 g
Cooking oil	1 tbsp.	15 mL
Medium peeled cooking apples (such as McIntosh), cut into 1/2 inch (12 mm) pieces	2	2
Ground cinnamon	1/8 tsp.	0.5 mL
Can of sweet potatoes, drained	19 oz.	540 mL
Brown sugar, packed	1 tsp.	5 mL
Ground ginger	1/4 tsp.	1 mL
Ground nutmeg	1/8 tsp.	0.5 mL
PECAN CRUMBLE TOPPING		
Brown sugar, packed	1/3 cup	75 mL
All-purpose flour	3 tbsp.	50 mL
Hard margarine (or butter)	3 tbsp.	50 mL
Chopped pecans	1/4 cup	60 mL

Combine first 4 ingredients in large resealable freezer bag. Add pork. Seal bag. Toss until coated.

Heat cooking oil in large frying pan on medium-high. Add pork. Cook for about 3 minutes, stirring often, until browned. Transfer with slotted spoon to ungreased 2 quart (2 L) shallow baking dish.

Heat and stir apple and cinnamon in same large frying pan for about 1 minute, scraping any brown bits from bottom of pan, until apple is tender-crisp. Add to pork. Stir. Spread evenly in baking dish.

Mash next 4 ingredients in large bowl until smooth. Spread evenly on top of pork mixture.

Pecan Crumble Topping: Combine brown sugar and flour in small bowl. Cut in margarine until mixture resembles fine crumbs. Add pecans. Stir. Makes about 3/4 cup (175 mL) topping. Sprinkle evenly over sweet potato mixture. Bake, uncovered, in 350°F (175°C) oven for about 30 minutes until heated through and topping is golden. Serves 4.

1 serving: 533 Calories; 22.8 g Total Fat (13.2 g Mono, 3.9 g Poly, 4.2 g Sat); 72 mg Cholesterol; 57 g Carbohydrate; 3 g Fibre; 26 g Protein; 273 mg Sodium

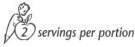

Chickpea Spinach Curry

Add a little colour to your day with this mild curry dish. Nice with rice.

Cooking oil	1 tbsp.	15 mL
Chopped onion	1 cup	250 mL
Curry powder	1 1/2 tbsp.	25 mL
Garlic cloves, minced	2	2
(or 1/2 tsp., 2 mL, powder)		
Cans of chickpeas (garbanzo beans),	2	2
19 oz. (540 mL) each, rinsed and		
drained		
Can of plum tomatoes (with juice)	28 oz.	796 mL
Cubed fresh peeled orange-fleshed	2 cups	500 mL
sweet potato		
Low-sodium prepared chicken broth	1/2 cup	125 mL
Granulated sugar	1/2 tsp.	2 mL
Garlic and herb no-salt seasoning (such	1/2 tsp.	2 mL
as Mrs. Dash)		
Pepper	1/4 tsp.	1 mL
Fresh spinach, stems removed,	2 cups	500 mL
lightly packed		
Low-fat plain yogurt	3 tbsp.	50 mL

Heat cooking oil in large pot or Dutch oven on medium. Add onion. Cook for 5 to 10 minutes, stirring often, until softened.

Add curry powder and garlic. Heat and stir for about 1 minute until fragrant.

Add next 7 ingredients. Stir. Bring to a boil on medium-high. Reduce heat to medium-low. Cover. Simmer for about 35 minutes, stirring occasionally, until sweet potato is tender.

Add spinach and yogurt. Stir. Cook for 1 to 2 minutes, stirring occasionally, until spinach is wilted. Serves 6.

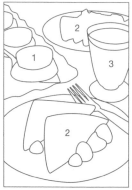

1 serving: 268 Calories; 5.1 g Total Fat (1.9 g Mono, 1.8 g Poly, 0.5 g Sat); 0 mg Cholesterol; 48 g Carbohydrate; 8 g Fibre; 11 g Protein; 491 mg Sodium

1. Potato Cakes Benny, page 62
2. Fruit-Full French Toast, page 65
3. Apricot Breakfast Drink, page 11

Props courtesy of: Emile Henry
Casa Bugatti
Klass Works

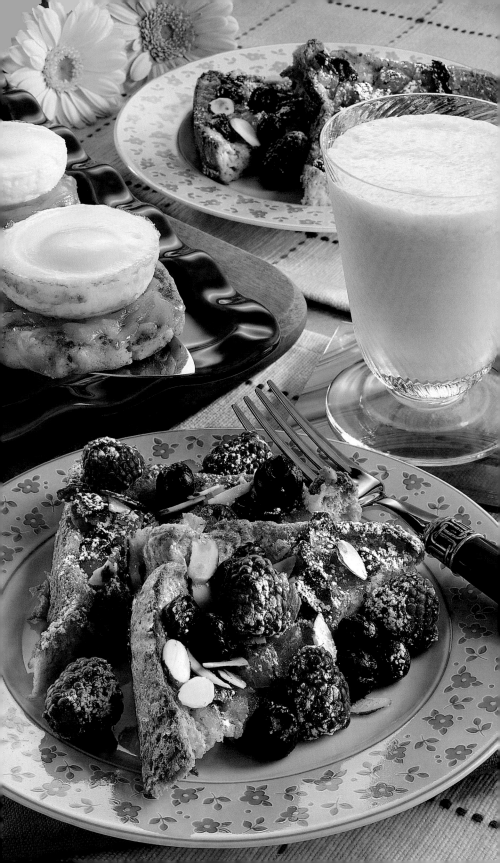

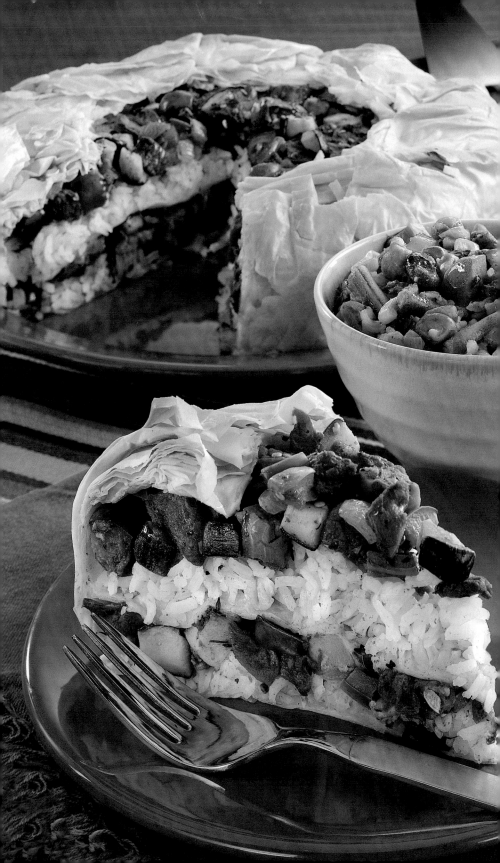

Stuffed Roasted Peppers

Plump, whole red peppers stuffed with delicious lentils and rice. A cheese and basil topping sprinkled over the stuffing adds a nice touch.

Large red peppers	4	4
Cooking oil	2 tsp.	10 mL
Finely chopped zucchini (with peel)	1 1/2 cups	375 mL
Finely chopped onion	1 cup	250 mL
Bacon slices, cooked crisp and crumbled	4	4
Can of brown lentils, rinsed and drained	19 oz.	540 mL
Can of diced tomatoes, drained and juice reserved	14 oz.	398 mL
Cooked brown rice (about 1/3 cup, 75 mL, uncooked)	1 cup	250 mL
Pepper	1/4 tsp.	1 mL
Grated Parmesan cheese	1/3 cup	75 mL
Chopped fresh basil (or 1 1/2 tsp., 7 mL, dried)	2 tbsp.	30 mL

Slice 1/2 inch (12 mm) from top of each red pepper. Set tops aside. Remove seeds and ribs. Trim bottom of each pepper so it will sit flat, being careful not to cut into cavity. Place peppers in greased 3 quart (3 L) casserole.

Heat cooking oil in large frying pan on medium. Add zucchini and onion. Cook for 5 to 10 minutes, stirring often, until onion is softened.

Add next 5 ingredients. Stir. Cook for about 5 minutes, stirring occasionally, until heated through. Spoon into prepared peppers. Replace tops. Pour reserved tomato juice over and around peppers in casserole. Bake, uncovered, in 350°F (175°C) oven for 35 to 40 minutes until peppers are tender-crisp.

Discard tops. Combine Parmesan cheese and basil in small bowl. Sprinkle over peppers. Serves 4.

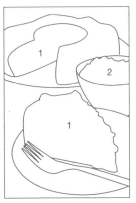

1 serving: 294 Calories; 6.9 g Total Fat (3.2 g Mono, 1.7 g Poly, 1.5 g Sat); 5 mg Cholesterol; 48 g Carbohydrate; 9 g Fibre; 14 g Protein; 444 mg Sodium

1. Ratatouille Pie, page 66
2. Calico Rice Creole, page 68

Props courtesy of: Cherison Enterprises Inc.
Danesco Inc.

Bean and Turkey Bake

This one's sure to be gobbled up quickly! Serve with rice or mashed potatoes.

Frozen French-style green beans	6 cups	1.5 L
Water		
Salt	1/2 tsp.	2 mL
Cooking oil	2 tsp.	10 mL
Lean ground turkey	1 lb.	454 g
Chopped onion	1/2 cup	125 mL
All-purpose flour	2 tsp.	10 mL
Can of condensed mushroom soup	10 oz.	284 mL
Low-sodium soy sauce	1 tsp.	5 mL
Fresh bean sprouts	3 cups	750 mL
Hard margarine (or butter)	2 tbsp.	30 mL
Fine dry bread crumbs	1/2 cup	125 mL

Cook green beans in water and salt in medium saucepan until tender-crisp. Drain. Cover to keep warm.

Heat cooking oil in large frying pan on medium-high. Add ground turkey and onion. Scramble-fry for 5 to 10 minutes until turkey is no longer pink.

Add flour. Stir. Add soup and soy sauce. Heat and stir for about 2 minutes until boiling.

Add green beans and bean sprouts. Stir. Spread evenly in ungreased 2 quart (2 L) shallow baking dish.

Melt margarine in small saucepan. Add bread crumbs. Mix well. Sprinkle evenly over turkey mixture. Bake, uncovered, in 350°F (175°C) oven for about 30 minutes until heated through and crumbs are golden. Serves 4.

1 serving: 467 Calories; 24.4 g Total Fat (10.1 g Mono, 6.6 g Poly, 5.7 g Sat); 90 mg Cholesterol; 36 g Carbohydrate; 5 g Fibre; 29 g Protein; 965 mg Sodium

BEAN AND CHICKEN BAKE: Omit lean ground turkey. Use same amount of lean ground chicken.

Leek and Potato Cod

No harm in letting the news "leek" out that dinner's cooking! Reel your family into the kitchen with the aroma of this zesty dilled dish.

Cooking oil	1 tbsp.	15 mL
Thinly sliced leek (white part only)	1 1/2 cups	375 mL
Thinly sliced red pepper	1 cup	250 mL
Thinly sliced baby potato	2 cups	500 mL
Low-sodium prepared chicken broth	1 1/2 cups	375 mL
Lemon juice	2 tbsp.	30 mL
Dijon mustard (with whole seeds)	2 tsp.	10 mL
Grated lemon zest	1 tsp.	5 mL
Cod fillets (about 1 lb., 454 g), any small bones removed	4	4
Chopped fresh dill (or 3/4 tsp., 4 mL, dried)	1 tbsp.	15 mL
Pepper, sprinkle		

Heat cooking oil in large frying pan on medium. Add leek and red pepper. Cook for 5 to 10 minutes, stirring often, until leek is softened. Spread evenly in frying pan.

Layer potato slices on top of leek mixture.

Combine next 4 ingredients in small bowl. Pour over potato. Cover. Cook for 8 to 10 minutes until potato is tender.

Place fillets in single layer on top of potato. Sprinkle with dill and pepper. Cover. Cook on medium-low for 8 to 10 minutes, depending on thickness of fillets, until fish flakes easily when tested with fork. Serves 4.

1 serving: 229 Calories; 4.7 g Total Fat (2.2 g Mono, 1.6 g Poly, 0.5 g Sat); 49 mg Cholesterol; 23 g Carbohydrate; 3 g Fibre; 24 g Protein; 355 mg Sodium

Squash Mushroom Lasagna

Sweet squash and carrots add a depth of flavour to earthy mushrooms in this scrumptious dish. Good cold too!

ONION CREAM SAUCE

Cooking oil	1 tsp.	5 mL
Chopped onion	1/2 cup	125 mL
Garlic cloves, minced	2	2
(or 1/2 tsp., 2 mL, powder)		
All-purpose flour	1/4 cup	60 mL
Can of skim evaporated milk	13 1/2 oz.	385 mL
Milk	1 cup	250 mL
Prepared vegetable broth	1/2 cup	125 mL
Sliced fresh white mushrooms	3 cups	750 mL
Grated carrot	1 cup	250 mL
Grated butternut squash	1 cup	250 mL
Lemon pepper	1 tsp.	5 mL
Dried oregano	1/2 tsp.	2 mL
1% cottage cheese	1 1/2 cups	375 mL
Grated Parmesan cheese	1/4 cup	60 mL
Large eggs	2	2
Oven-ready lasagna noodles	9	9
Grated part-skim mozzarella cheese	1 cup	250 mL
Chopped fresh parsley, for garnish	2 tbsp.	30 mL

Onion Cream Sauce: Heat cooking oil in medium saucepan on medium. Add onion and garlic. Cook for 5 to 10 minutes, stirring often, until onion is softened.

Add flour. Heat and stir for 1 minute. Slowly add evaporated milk and milk, stirring constantly. Heat and stir for 5 to 10 minutes until boiling and thickened. Remove from heat. Makes about 2 1/2 cups (625 mL) cream sauce. Set aside.

Measure broth into large frying pan. Bring to a boil on medium-high. Add mushrooms. Heat and stir for 2 minutes.

Add next 4 ingredients. Cook, uncovered, for 5 to 10 minutes, stirring often, until liquid is evaporated. Remove from heat. Let stand for 10 minutes.

Add next 3 ingredients. Stir well.

(continued on next page)

Layer ingredients in greased 9 x 13 inch (22 x 33 cm) pan as follows:

1. 1/2 cup (125 mL) Onion Cream Sauce, spread evenly in pan

2. 3 noodles

3. Half of vegetable mixture

4. 2/3 cup (150 mL) cream sauce

5. 3 noodles

6. Remaining vegetable mixture

7. 2/3 cup (150 mL) cream sauce

8. Remaining noodles

9. Remaining cream sauce, spread evenly on top

Sprinkle with mozzarella cheese. Cover with greased foil. Bake in 350°F (175°C) oven for 45 minutes. Discard foil. Bake for about 15 minutes until noodles are tender and mozzarella cheese is golden. Let stand for 15 minutes.

Garnish with parsley. Cuts into 8 pieces.

1 piece: 251 Calories; 6.7 g Total Fat (2.1 g Mono, 0.6 g Poly, 3.3 g Sat); 71 mg Cholesterol; 27 g Carbohydrate; 2 g Fibre; 21 g Protein; 548 mg Sodium

Paré Pointer

Photos of Abe Lincoln always show him standing up because he would never lie.

Shrimp and Asparagus Pasta

A feast for the eyes before you even lift a fork. Serve with a crisp salad.

Fettuccine	13 oz.	370 g
Boiling water	10 cups	2.5 L
Salt	1 1/4 tsp.	6 mL
Olive (or cooking) oil	1 tbsp.	15 mL
Chopped red onion	1 cup	250 mL
Can of diced tomatoes, drained	14 oz.	398 mL
Granulated sugar	1/2 tsp.	2 mL
Salt	1/4 tsp.	1 mL
Pepper	1/4 tsp.	1 mL
Fresh asparagus, trimmed of tough ends and cut into 1 inch (2.5 cm) pieces	1/2 lb.	225 g
Uncooked medium shrimp (peeled and deveined)	1 lb.	454 g
Chopped fresh parsley	2 tbsp.	30 mL
Grated Parmesan cheese (optional)	2 tbsp.	30 mL
Lemon juice	1 tbsp.	15 mL

Cook fettuccine in boiling water and salt in large uncovered pot or Dutch oven for 12 to 15 minutes, stirring occasionally, until tender but firm. Drain. Return to same pot. Cover to keep warm.

Heat olive oil in large frying pan on medium. Add onion. Cook for 5 to 10 minutes, stirring often, until softened.

Add next 4 ingredients. Stir. Bring to a boil.

Add asparagus. Stir. Cook for about 3 minutes until asparagus is almost tender-crisp.

Add shrimp. Stir. Cook for about 2 minutes until shrimp turn pink and asparagus is tender-crisp. Add to fettuccine.

Add remaining 3 ingredients. Toss gently. Remove to large serving dish. Serves 4.

1 serving: 520 Calories; 6.8 g Total Fat (3 g Mono, 1.6 g Poly, 1 g Sat); 129 mg Cholesterol; 82 g Carbohydrate; 5 g Fibre; 32 g Protein; 449 mg Sodium

Pictured on page 89.

Eggplant Pasta Bake

Whole-wheat pasta adds a nutty flavour to this rich, tomatoey dish. Scrumptious.

Whole-wheat penne (or other tube) pasta	2 cups	500 mL
Boiling water	10 cups	2.5 L
Salt	1 1/4 tsp.	6 mL
Eggplant, peeled and cut lengthwise into 1/4 inch (6 mm) slices	2	2
Salt, sprinkle		
Olive (or cooking) oil	1 tbsp.	15 mL
Chopped onion	1 cup	250 mL
Pasta sauce	2 3/4 cups	675 mL
Roma (plum) tomatoes, chopped	6	6
Basil pesto	1/4 cup	60 mL
Grated Parmesan cheese	1/2 cup	125 mL
Grated part-skim mozzarella cheese	1/2 cup	125 mL

Cook pasta in boiling water and salt in large uncovered pot or Dutch oven for 10 to 12 minutes, stirring occasionally, until tender but firm. Drain. Return to same pot. Cover to keep warm.

Sprinkle both sides of each eggplant slice with salt. Place on wire rack set in baking sheet with sides. Let stand for 20 minutes. Rinse slices with cold water. Pat dry with paper towels. Spray both sides of each slice with cooking spray. Preheat electric grill for 5 minutes or gas barbecue to medium (see Note). Cook slices on greased grill for 2 to 3 minutes per side until golden. Transfer to large plate. Cut into 1 inch (2.5 cm) pieces.

Heat olive oil in large frying pan on medium. Add onion. Cook for 5 to 10 minutes, stirring often, until softened.

Add eggplant, pasta and next 3 ingredients. Stir well. Spread evenly in greased 3 quart (3 L) casserole.

Sprinkle with both cheeses. Bake, uncovered, in 350°F (175°C) oven for 30 to 40 minutes until heated through and cheese is golden. Serves 6.

1 serving: 413 Calories; 16.5 g Total Fat (8.3 g Mono, 2.6 g Poly, 4.5 g Sat); 13 mg Cholesterol; 57 g Carbohydrate; 10 g Fibre; 15 g Protein; 829 mg Sodium

Note: If preferred, cook eggplant slices in 3 batches in 1 tbsp. (15 mL) olive (or cooking) oil in large frying pan on medium for 3 to 5 minutes per side until golden.

Broccoli Macaroni Bake

Macaroni and cheese that's fancy enough for company. This one will soon be a favourite!

Broccoli florets	4 cups	1 L
Boiling water		
Ice water		
Elbow macaroni	1 1/2 cups	375 mL
Boiling water	8 cups	2 L
Salt	1 tsp.	5 mL
Hard margarine (or butter)	1 tbsp.	15 mL
Finely chopped onion	1 cup	250 mL
Chopped red pepper	1 cup	250 mL
Chopped low-fat deli ham	1 cup	250 mL
All-purpose flour	1/3 cup	75 mL
Milk	4 cups	1 L
Grated light sharp Cheddar cheese	2 cups	500 mL
Chopped fresh parsley	1/4 cup	60 mL
Dijon mustard	2 tsp.	10 mL
Garlic and herb (or Italian) no-salt seasoning (such as Mrs. Dash)	1 tsp.	5 mL
Pepper	1/4 tsp.	1 mL
Hard margarine (or butter)	1 tbsp.	15 mL
Fine dry bread crumbs	1/4 cup	60 mL

Cook broccoli in boiling water in large saucepan for about 5 minutes until bright green. Drain. Immediately plunge into ice water in large bowl. Let stand for about 10 minutes until cold. Drain. Set aside.

Cook macaroni in boiling water and salt in large uncovered pot or Dutch oven for 8 to 10 minutes, stirring occasionally, until tender but firm. Drain. Transfer to medium bowl. Set aside.

Melt first amount of margarine in same large pot on medium. Add next 3 ingredients. Cook for 5 to 10 minutes, stirring often, until onion is softened.

Add flour. Heat and stir for 1 minute. Slowly add milk, stirring constantly. Heat and stir for 5 to 10 minutes until boiling and thickened. Remove from heat.

Add next 5 ingredients. Stir until cheese is melted. Add broccoli and macaroni. Stir until coated. Spread evenly in greased 2 1/2 quart (2.5 L) casserole.

(continued on next page)

Melt second amount of margarine in small saucepan on medium. Add bread crumbs. Mix well. Sprinkle over top of macaroni mixture. Bake in 350°F (175°C) oven for about 30 minutes until heated through. Serves 6.

1 serving: 487 Calories; 21.4 g Total Fat (7.6 g Mono, 1.5 g Poly, 10.9 g Sat); 60 mg Cholesterol; 47 g Carbohydrate; 4 g Fibre; 28 g Protein; 825 mg Sodium

(2) *servings per portion*

Zucchini Tomato Spaghetti

Feta and garlic add a delightful nip to this simple pasta dish. Serve with warm rolls.

Whole-wheat spaghetti	13 oz.	370 g
Boiling water	10 cups	2.5 L
Salt	1 1/4 tsp.	6 mL
Olive (or cooking) oil	1 tbsp.	15 mL
Medium zucchini (with peel), chopped	4	4
Garlic cloves, minced	2	2
(or 1/2 tsp., 2 mL, powder)		
Roma (plum) tomatoes, quartered	4	4
lengthwise		
Light feta cheese, cubed	4 1/2 oz.	125 g
Chopped fresh parsley	1/4 cup	60 mL
Lemon juice	1 tbsp.	15 mL
Pepper	1/4 tsp.	1 mL

Cook spaghetti in boiling water and salt in large uncovered pot or Dutch oven for 10 to 12 minutes, stirring occasionally, until tender but firm. Drain. Return to same pot. Cover to keep warm.

Heat olive oil in large frying pan on medium. Add zucchini and garlic. Cook for 5 to 10 minutes, stirring occasionally, until zucchini is softened.

Add tomato. Heat and stir for about 3 minutes until tomato just starts to soften. Add to spaghetti.

Add remaining 4 ingredients. Toss gently. Serves 6.

1 serving: 328 Calories; 8.2 g Total Fat (2.9 g Mono, 0.8 g Poly, 3.8 g Sat); 19 mg Cholesterol; 55 g Carbohydrate; 8 g Fibre; 14 g Protein; 257 mg Sodium

Creamy Mushroom Pasta

Tender pasta snuggles with earthy mushrooms, smoky ham and sweet peas in a creamy, cheesy sauce. Delicious!

Package of dried porcini mushrooms	3/4 oz.	22 g
Boiling water		
Medium bow (or other) pasta	1 1/2 cups	375 mL
Boiling water	8 cups	2 L
Salt	1 tsp.	5 mL
Cooking oil	1 tbsp.	15 mL
Sliced fresh brown (or white) mushrooms	3 cups	750 mL
Chopped low-fat deli ham	1 cup	250 mL
All-purpose flour	2 tbsp.	30 mL
Milk	2 cups	500 mL
Low-sodium prepared chicken broth	1/2 cup	125 mL
Dijon mustard	1 tbsp.	15 mL
Pepper	1/4 tsp.	1 mL
Frozen peas	1 cup	250 mL
Chopped fresh parsley	1/4 cup	60 mL
Grated light sharp Cheddar cheese	2/3 cup	150 mL

Put porcini mushrooms into small bowl. Pour boiling water over top until covered. Let stand for about 20 minutes until softened. Drain. Rinse with cold water. Squeeze to remove excess liquid. Discard stems. Thinly slice caps.

Cook pasta in boiling water and salt in large uncovered pot or Dutch oven for 12 to 15 minutes, stirring occasionally, until tender but firm. Drain. Return to same pot. Cover to keep warm.

Heat cooking oil in large frying pan on medium-high. Add porcini mushrooms, brown mushrooms and ham. Stir. Cook for about 5 minutes, stirring occasionally, until mushrooms start to brown.

Add flour. Heat and stir for 1 minute. Slowly add next 4 ingredients. Heat and stir for about 5 minutes until boiling and thickened.

Add peas and parsley. Heat and stir for about 5 minutes until peas are heated through. Remove from heat.

Add cheese. Stir until melted. Add to pasta. Stir until coated. Serves 4.

1 serving: 503 Calories; 14.4 g Total Fat (5.7 g Mono, 2.3 g Poly, 5.1 g Sat); 39 mg Cholesterol; 65 g Carbohydrate; 5 g Fibre; 28 g Protein; 870 mg Sodium

Tomato and Chickpea Pasta

Bright red tomato and deep green spinach make this meatless pasta dish an attractive entree. A hearty meal.

Medium bow (or other) pasta	2 1/2 cups	625 mL
Boiling water	10 cups	2.5 L
Salt	1 1/4 tsp.	6 mL
Olive (or cooking) oil	1 tbsp.	15 mL
Cherry tomatoes, halved	12 oz.	340 g
Chili paste (sambal oelek)	1/2 tsp.	2 mL
Garlic cloves, minced (or 1/2 tsp., 2 mL, powder)	2	2
Can of chickpeas (garbanzo beans), rinsed and drained	19 oz.	540 mL
Fresh spinach, stems removed, lightly packed	3 cups	750 mL
Crumbled light feta cheese	3/4 cup	175 mL

Cook pasta in boiling water and salt in large uncovered pot or Dutch oven for 12 to 15 minutes, stirring occasionally, until tender but firm. Drain. Return to same pot. Cover to keep warm.

Heat olive oil in large frying pan on medium. Add next 3 ingredients. Heat and stir for about 2 minutes until fragrant.

Add chickpeas and spinach. Heat and stir for 3 to 4 minutes until spinach is wilted. Add to pasta. Toss.

Add cheese. Toss well. Serves 4.

1 serving: 414 Calories; 13 g Total Fat (4.5 g Mono, 1.6 g Poly, 5.6 g Sat); 29 mg Cholesterol; 58 g Carbohydrate; 6 g Fibre; 18 g Protein; 550 mg Sodium

Paré Pointer

A horse and an egg both have to be broken to use.

Pepper Mushroom Ravioli

Mushrooms, colourful peppers and a white wine cream sauce perfectly complement tender ravioli.

Cooking oil	1 tbsp.	15 mL
Sliced fresh white mushrooms	2 cups	500 mL
Chopped red pepper	1 cup	250 mL
Chopped yellow pepper	1 cup	250 mL
Garlic cloves, minced	2	2
(or 1/2 tsp., 2 mL, powder)		
Dry (or alcohol-free) white wine	1/3 cup	75 mL
Low-sodium prepared chicken	1/3 cup	75 mL
(or vegetable) broth		
Light sour cream	2 tbsp.	30 mL
Finely shredded fresh basil	2 tbsp.	30 mL
(or 1 1/2 tsp., 7 mL, dried)		
Pepper	1/4 tsp.	1 mL
Package of fresh cheese (or your favourite) ravioli	10 1/2 oz.	300 g
Shaved Parmesan cheese	1/3 cup	75 mL

Heat cooking oil in large frying pan on medium. Add next 4 ingredients. Cook for 5 to 10 minutes, stirring occasionally, until peppers are softened.

Add wine. Stir. Bring to a boil. Boil gently for about 5 minutes, stirring occasionally, until wine is almost evaporated.

Add broth. Bring to a boil. Add next 3 ingredients. Stir. Reduce heat to low. Cover to keep warm.

Cook ravioli according to package directions. Drain. Add to mushroom mixture. Stir until coated. Spoon onto each of 4 plates.

Scatter Parmesan cheese over each. Serves 4.

1 serving: 283 Calories; 13.3 g Total Fat (3.1 g Mono, 1.3 g Poly, 2.6 g Sat); 53 mg Cholesterol; 24 g Carbohydrate; 2 g Fibre; 15 g Protein; 415 mg Sodium

Sun-Dried Tomato Frittata

A delicious weekend brunch. Great with toast and juice.

Penne (or other tube) pasta	1 1/2 cups	375 mL
Boiling water	8 cups	2 L
Salt	1 tsp.	5 mL
Cooking oil	1 tbsp.	15 mL
Medium zucchini (with peel), chopped	2	2
Finely chopped onion	1 cup	250 mL
Sun-dried tomatoes in oil, blotted dry, chopped	1/2 cup	125 mL
Chopped fresh thyme leaves (or 1/4 tsp., 1 mL, dried)	1 1/2 tsp.	7 mL
Pepper	1/4 tsp.	1 mL
Large eggs	8	8
Milk	1/4 cup	60 mL
Grated Parmesan cheese	1 tbsp.	15 mL
Grated sharp white Cheddar cheese	3/4 cup	175 mL

Cook pasta in boiling water and salt in large uncovered pot or Dutch oven for 10 to 12 minutes, stirring occasionally, until tender but firm. Drain. Return to same pot. Cover to keep warm.

Heat cooking oil in large frying pan on medium. Add zucchini and onion. Cook for 5 to 10 minutes, stirring often, until onion is softened.

Add pasta and next 3 ingredients. Heat and stir for about 5 minutes until heated through. Spread evenly in pan.

Beat next 3 ingredients with whisk in medium bowl. Pour over pasta mixture. Reduce heat to medium-low. Cover. Cook for 3 to 5 minutes until bottom is golden and top is almost set. Remove cover.

Sprinkle with Cheddar cheese. Broil 4 inches (10 cm) from heat in oven (see Note) for about 2 minutes until Cheddar cheese is melted and frittata is set. Cuts into 8 wedges. Serves 4.

1 serving: 547 Calories; 24.7 g Total Fat (9.5 g Mono, 3.3 g Poly, 8.9 g Sat); 456 mg Cholesterol; 53 g Carbohydrate; 4 g Fibre; 28 g Protein; 349 mg Sodium

Note: To avoid damaging frying pan handle in oven, wrap handle with foil before placing under broiler.

Spicy Sweet Chicken Stew

Sweet raisins and dates mingle nicely in this spicy curry stew. Lots of sauce to serve over potatoes, noodles or rice.

All-purpose flour	3 tbsp.	50 mL
Bone-in chicken thighs, skin removed	1 3/4 lbs.	790 g
Cooking oil	1 tbsp.	15 mL
Thinly sliced onion	1 cup	250 mL
Cinnamon stick (4 inches, 10 cm)	1	1
Ground cumin	2 tsp.	10 mL
Ground coriander	2 tsp.	10 mL
Turmeric	1/2 tsp.	2 mL
Pepper	1/2 tsp.	2 mL
Low-sodium prepared chicken broth	3 cups	750 mL
Medium carrots, cut into 1/4 inch (6 mm) pieces	2	2
Medium red pepper, seeds and ribs removed, cut into 1/4 inch (6 mm) pieces	1	1
Medium zucchini (with peel), cut into 1/4 inch (6 mm) pieces	2	2
Medium tomatoes, peeled (see Tip, page 38), chopped	2	2
Dark raisins	1 cup	250 mL
Chopped pitted dates	1/2 cup	125 mL
Water	1/4 cup	60 mL
All-purpose flour	2 tbsp.	30 mL

Measure first amount of flour into large resealable freezer bag. Add chicken. Seal bag. Toss until coated.

Heat cooking oil in large pot or Dutch oven on medium. Add chicken. Cook for 3 to 4 minutes per side until browned. Transfer to large plate. Cover to keep warm.

Cook onion in same large pot for 5 to 10 minutes, stirring often, until softened.

Add next 5 ingredients. Heat and stir for about 1 minute until fragrant.

(continued on next page)

Slowly add broth, stirring constantly and scraping any brown bits from bottom of pot. Add chicken, carrot and red pepper. Stir. Bring to a boil. Reduce heat to medium-low. Cover. Simmer for 15 minutes. Increase heat to medium. Cook, uncovered, for 10 to 15 minutes until chicken is no longer pink inside.

Add next 4 ingredients. Stir. Cook for about 10 minutes, stirring occasionally, until vegetables are tender-crisp and raisins and dates are softened. Discard cinnamon stick. Transfer chicken and vegetables with slotted spoon to large serving bowl. Cover to keep warm. Bring broth mixture to a boil.

Stir water into second amount of flour in small cup until smooth. Slowly add to broth mixture, stirring constantly. Heat and stir for 2 to 3 minutes until boiling and thickened. Spoon onto chicken and vegetables. Serves 6.

1 serving: 332 Calories; 7.7 g Total Fat (2.9 g Mono, 2 g Poly, 1.4 g Sat); 69 mg Cholesterol; 49 g Carbohydrate; 6 g Fibre; 21 g Protein; 340 mg Sodium

Pictured on page 90.

 tip
If a recipe calls for less than an entire can of tomato paste, freeze unopened can for 30 minutes. Open both ends and push contents through one end. Slice off only what you need. Freeze remaining paste in resealable freezer bag or plastic wrap for future use.

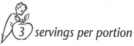

Curried Pork Stew

A medley of chunky vegetables smothered in a thick, spicy sauce. Its wonderful aroma will make everyone scurry to the curry in a hurry to eat!

Cooking oil	1 tbsp.	15 mL
Stewing pork	1 lb.	454 g
Curry powder	1 1/2 tbsp.	25 mL
Chopped carrot	2 cups	500 mL
Chopped onion	1 1/2 cups	375 mL
Low-sodium prepared chicken broth	1 1/2 cups	375 mL
Chopped yellow turnip (rutabaga)	1 cup	250 mL
Chopped celery	1/2 cup	125 mL
Tomato paste (see Tip, page 87)	1/4 cup	60 mL
Bay leaves	2	2
Pepper	1/4 tsp.	1 mL

Heat cooking oil in large pot or Dutch oven on medium. Add pork. Cook for about 10 minutes, stirring occasionally, until browned.

Add curry powder. Heat and stir for about 1 minute until fragrant.

Add remaining 8 ingredients. Stir. Bring to a boil on medium-high. Reduce heat to medium-low. Cover. Simmer for about 1 hour, stirring occasionally, until pork is tender. Remove cover. Bring to a boil on medium. Boil gently for about 10 minutes until sauce is thickened. Discard bay leaves. Serves 4.

1 serving: 400 Calories; 24.7 g Total Fat (11.2 g Mono, 3.4 g Poly, 7.4 g Sat); 81 mg Cholesterol; 22 g Carbohydrate; 5 g Fibre; 24 g Protein; 419 mg Sodium

1. Shrimp and Asparagus Pasta, page 78
2. Minted Beef and Noodles, page 46

Props courtesy of: Pfaltzgraff Canada
Klass Works
Casa Bugatti
Totally Bamboo

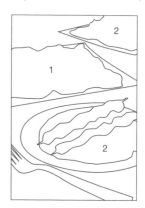

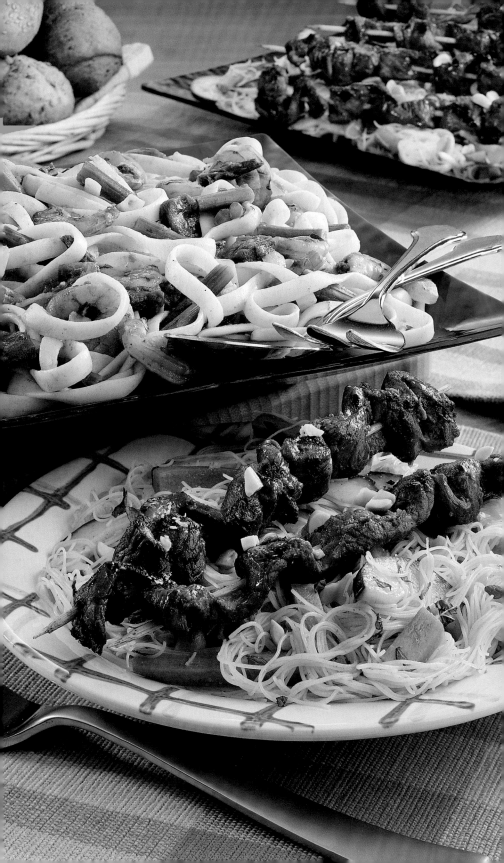

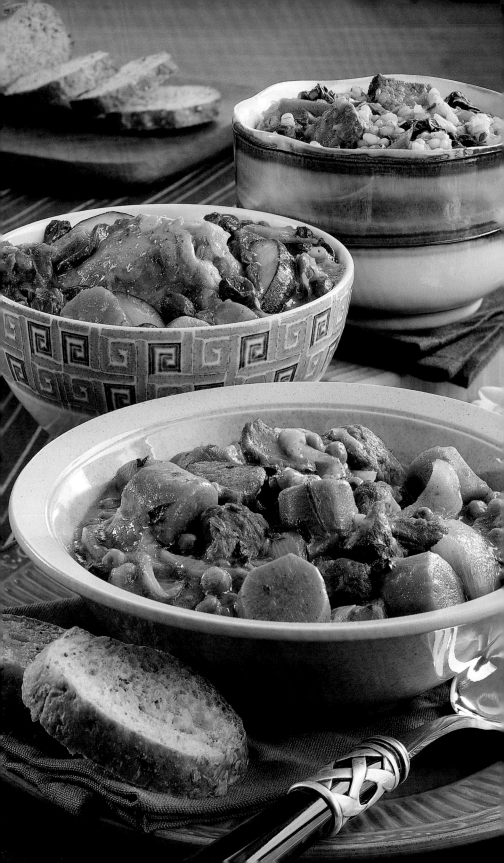

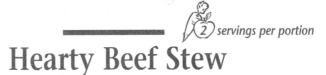
Hearty Beef Stew

Rich, dark and delicious. Serve with thick bread slices or crusty rolls. Equally good over egg noodles.

Cooking oil	1 tbsp.	15 mL
Stewing beef	1 1/2 lbs.	680 g
Can of diced tomatoes (with juice)	28 oz.	796 mL
Chopped onion	1 1/2 cups	375 mL
Chopped carrot	1 1/2 cups	375 mL
Chopped parsnip	1 cup	250 mL
Dry (or alcohol-free) red wine	3/4 cup	175 mL
Chopped celery	1/2 cup	125 mL
Worcestershire sauce	1 tbsp.	15 mL
Garlic and herb no-salt seasoning (such as Mrs. Dash)	1/2 tsp.	2 mL
Bay leaves	2	2
Pepper	1/2 tsp.	2 mL
Water	3 tbsp.	50 mL
All-purpose flour	3 tbsp.	50 mL

Heat cooking oil in large frying pan on medium-high. Add beef in 2 batches. Cook for about 7 minutes per batch, stirring occasionally, until browned. Transfer to greased 3 quart (3 L) casserole.

Add next 10 ingredients. Stir. Cover. Cook in 325°F (160°C) oven for about 1 1/2 hours until vegetables are softened and beef is almost tender.

Stir water into flour in small cup until smooth. Slowly add to beef mixture, stirring constantly. Return to oven. Cook, uncovered, for about 30 minutes, stirring once, until beef is tender and sauce is boiling and thickened. Serves 6.

1 serving: 322 Calories; 12.1 g Total Fat (5.4 g Mono, 1.3 g Poly, 4 g Sat); 59 mg Cholesterol; 22 g Carbohydrate; 4 g Fibre; 26 g Protein; 355 mg Sodium

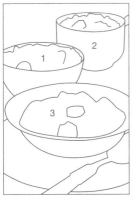

1. Spicy Sweet Chicken Stew, page 86
2. Barley Beef Stew, page 99
3. Minted Lamb and Pea Braise, page 94

Props courtesy of: Mikasa Home Store
                           Totally Bamboo
                           Casa Bugatti
                           Winners

Roasted Pepper Goulash

Deliciously tender pork with mellow roasted peppers in lots of creamy sauce. Serve over egg noodles.

Large green pepper	1	1
Large red pepper	1	1
Large orange (or yellow) pepper	1	1
All-purpose flour	1/3 cup	75 mL
Garlic and herb no-salt seasoning (such as Mrs. Dash)	2 tsp.	10 mL
Lemon pepper	1 tsp.	5 mL
Boneless pork loin roast, cut into 1/4 inch (6 mm) slices, then into thin strips	1 1/2 lbs.	680 g
Cooking oil	3 tbsp.	50 mL
Large onion, thinly sliced	1	1
Garlic clove, minced (or 1/4 tsp., 1 mL, powder)	1	1
Water	1/3 cup	75 mL
Paprika	2 tbsp.	30 mL
Can of diced tomatoes (with juice)	14 oz.	398 mL
Can of condensed vegetable broth	10 oz.	284 mL
Granulated sugar	1 tsp.	5 mL
Garlic and herb no-salt seasoning (such as Mrs. Dash)	1/2 tsp.	2 mL
Light sour cream	1 cup	250 mL
All-purpose flour	2 tbsp.	30 mL
Finely chopped fresh parsley (or 1 1/2 tsp., 7 mL, flakes)	2 tbsp.	30 mL

Place peppers on ungreased baking sheet. Broil 4 inches (10 cm) from heat in oven for about 10 minutes, turning often, until skins are blistered and blackened. Transfer to large bowl. Cover with plastic wrap. Let stand for about 15 minutes until cool enough to handle. Remove skins. Cut peppers in half. Discard seeds and ribs, reserving any liquid. Strain liquid through sieve into small bowl. Cut peppers into strips. Set aside.

Measure next 3 ingredients into large resealable freezer bag. Add pork. Seal bag. Toss until coated.

(continued on next page)

Heat cooking oil in large pot or Dutch oven on medium-high. Cook pork in 2 batches for 5 to 10 minutes per batch, stirring often, until browned. Transfer with slotted spoon to paper towels to drain.

Combine next 3 ingredients in same large pot. Cook on medium for about 5 minutes, stirring often and scraping any brown bits from bottom of pot, until onion is softened.

Add paprika. Stir. Add pork, reserved liquid from peppers and next 4 ingredients. Stir. Reduce heat to medium-low. Cover. Simmer for about 1 1/2 hours, stirring occasionally, until pork is tender.

Beat sour cream and second amount of flour with whisk in small bowl until smooth. Add small amount of hot pork mixture. Stir well. Add to pork mixture in pot. Stir well.

Add pepper strips and parsley. Heat and stir on medium for about 5 minutes until sauce is boiling and slightly thickened. Serves 6.

1 serving: 430 Calories; 26.1 g Total Fat (12.9 g Mono, 4.5 g Poly, 9.2 g Sat); 79 mg Cholesterol; 22 g Carbohydrate; 3 g Fibre; 27 g Protein; 444 mg Sodium

---

Paré Pointer

Take away one lamp from the post and it becomes a lamplighter.

Minted Lamb and Pea Braise

A traditional combination, simmered to minty perfection in a succulent stew.

Stewing lamb	1 lb.	454 g
All-purpose flour	2 tbsp.	30 mL
Cooking oil	1 tbsp.	15 mL
Cooking oil	1 tsp.	5 mL
Small onions, quartered	2	2
Small carrots, cut into 3/4 inch (2 cm) pieces	4	4
Spiced apple cider	1 cup	250 mL
Frozen peas	1 cup	250 mL
Chopped fresh mint leaves	1/4 cup	60 mL

Put lamb into large resealable freezer bag. Add flour. Seal bag. Toss until coated.

Heat first amount of cooking oil in large saucepan on medium-high. Cook lamb in 2 batches for 5 to 6 minutes per batch, stirring occasionally, until browned. Transfer to medium bowl. Cover to keep warm.

Heat second amount of cooking oil in same large saucepan on medium. Add onion. Cook for 5 to 10 minutes, stirring often, until softened.

Add lamb, carrot and apple cider. Stir. Bring to a boil on medium-high. Reduce heat to medium-low. Cover. Simmer for about 1 1/2 hours, stirring occasionally, until lamb is tender. Remove cover. Bring to a boil on medium. Boil gently for about 5 minutes, stirring occasionally, until sauce is thickened.

Add peas and mint. Stir. Reduce heat to medium-low. Simmer, uncovered, for about 5 minutes until peas are heated through. Serves 4.

1 serving: 408 Calories; 24.4 g Total Fat (10.7 g Mono, 3.1 g Poly, 8.8 g Sat); 78 mg Cholesterol; 23 g Carbohydrate; 4 g Fibre; 24 g Protein; 130 mg Sodium

Pictured on page 90.

Mediterranean Hot Pot

A colourful dish with a full-bodied rosemary and tomato sauce that everyone's sure to love.

Cooking oil	1 tbsp.	15 mL
Boneless, skinless chicken thighs, halved	1 lb.	454 g
Bacon slices, cooked crisp and crumbled	4	4
Can of diced tomatoes (with juice)	28 oz.	796 mL
Chopped red onion	1 cup	250 mL
Chopped red pepper	1 cup	250 mL
Sprigs of fresh rosemary	2	2
Garlic cloves, minced	2	2
(or 1/2 tsp., 2 mL, powder)		
Granulated sugar	1/2 tsp.	2 mL
Pepper	1/4 tsp.	1 mL
Chopped kalamata olives	1/4 cup	60 mL
Cubed light feta cheese	1 1/2 oz.	43 g
Chopped fresh parsley	2 tbsp.	30 mL
(or 1 1/2 tsp., 7 mL, flakes)		

Heat cooking oil in large pot or Dutch oven on medium-high. Add chicken. Cook for 5 to 10 minutes, turning occasionally, until browned.

Add next 8 ingredients. Stir. Bring to a boil. Reduce heat to medium-low. Cover. Simmer for about 30 minutes, stirring occasionally, until chicken is no longer pink inside.

Add olives. Stir. Simmer, uncovered, for 1 to 2 minutes until heated through. Discard rosemary sprigs.

Sprinkle with cheese and parsley. Do not stir. Cover. Simmer for about 2 minutes until cheese is softened. Serves 4.

1 serving: 345 Calories; 18.1 g Total Fat (6.9 g Mono, 3.4 g Poly, 6 g Sat); 117 mg Cholesterol; 17 g Carbohydrate; 3 g Fibre; 29 g Protein; 698 mg Sodium

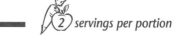

Pork and Apricot Braise

Deliciously sweet apricot sauce makes this stew fancy enough for company. Beautiful colour and a hint of spiciness—it's sure to satisfy.

Cooking oil	1 tbsp.	15 mL
Stewing pork	1 lb.	454 g
Ground cumin	2 tsp.	10 mL
Ground ginger	1 tsp.	5 mL
Dried crushed chilies	1/2 tsp.	2 mL
Chopped carrot	2 cups	500 mL
Low-sodium prepared chicken broth	1 cup	250 mL
Water	1 cup	250 mL
Chopped celery	1/2 cup	125 mL
Chopped dried apricot	1/2 cup	125 mL
Dry onion soup mix, stir before measuring	3 tbsp.	50 mL
Frozen peas	1 cup	250 mL
Chopped fresh parsley	3 tbsp.	50 mL
(or 2 1/4 tsp., 11 mL, flakes)		
Liquid honey	2 tbsp.	30 mL
Grated orange zest	1/2 tsp.	2 mL
Water (or orange juice)	2 tbsp.	30 mL
Cornstarch	1 tbsp.	15 mL

Heat cooking oil in large pot or Dutch oven on medium. Add pork. Cook for about 15 minutes, stirring occasionally, until browned.

Add next 3 ingredients. Heat and stir for about 1 minute until fragrant.

Add next 6 ingredients. Stir. Bring to a boil. Reduce heat to medium-low. Cover. Simmer for about 1 1/2 hours, stirring occasionally, until pork and carrot are tender.

Add next 4 ingredients. Stir. Bring to a boil on medium.

Stir water into cornstarch in small cup until smooth. Add to pork mixture. Heat and stir for 1 to 2 minutes until peas are tender-crisp and sauce is boiling and thickened. Serves 4.

1 serving: 494 Calories; 25.3 g Total Fat (11.6 g Mono, 3.5 g Poly, 7.6 g Sat); 81 mg Cholesterol; 43 g Carbohydrate; 6 g Fibre; 26 g Protein; 1361 mg Sodium

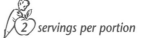

Sausage Ragout

A delightful tomato-based dish with plenty of spicy sausage and tender vegetables.
Serve with fresh brown bread to soak up the sauce.

Hot Italian sausages	1 lb.	454 g
Cooking oil	1 tsp.	5 mL
Chopped onion	1 cup	250 mL
Finely grated ginger root	1 tbsp.	15 mL
(or 3/4 tsp., 4 mL, ground)		
Garlic cloves, minced	2	2
(or 1/2 tsp., 2 mL, powder)		
Paprika	2 tsp.	10 mL
Dried crushed chilies	1/2 tsp.	2 mL
Ground cinnamon	1/4 tsp.	1 mL
Sliced carrot	1 1/2 cups	375 mL
Diced peeled potato	1 1/2 cups	375 mL
Low-sodium prepared chicken broth	2 cups	500 mL
Can of mixed beans, rinsed and drained	19 oz.	540 mL
Tomato sauce	1 cup	250 mL
Chopped fresh basil	2 tbsp.	30 mL

Randomly poke several holes with fork into each sausage. Heat cooking oil in large pot or Dutch oven on medium. Add sausages. Cook for about 10 minutes, turning occasionally, until browned. Transfer to paper towel-lined plate. Cover to keep warm. Discard drippings, reserving about 1 tbsp. (15 mL) in pot.

Add onion. Cook for 5 to 10 minutes, stirring often, until softened. Add next 5 ingredients. Heat and stir for about 1 minute until fragrant.

Add carrot and potato. Heat and stir on medium-high for 1 minute. Slowly add broth, stirring constantly and scraping any brown bits from bottom of pot. Add sausages. Bring to a boil. Reduce heat to medium-low. Cover. Simmer for about 10 minutes until carrot is almost tender. Transfer sausages with slotted spoon to cutting board. Cut into 1/2 inch (12 mm) slices. Return to carrot mixture.

Add beans and tomato sauce. Stir. Cook on medium-high for about 5 minutes, stirring occasionally, until sauce is boiling and thickened.

Add basil. Heat and stir for 1 minute to blend flavours. Serves 4.

1 serving: 425 Calories; 19.4 g Total Fat (8.7 g Mono, 3 g Poly, 6.4 g Sat); 45 mg Cholesterol; 44 g Carbohydrate; 8 g Fibre; 21 g Protein; 1402 mg Sodium

Chicken Vegetable Hot Pot

Rich, earthy flavours and wholesome vegetables abound in this sweet 'n' spicy stew.

Chinese dried mushrooms	8	8
Boiling water		
Water	1 tbsp.	15 mL
Cornstarch	1 tbsp.	15 mL
Cooking oil	2 tsp.	10 mL
Medium onion, cut into thin wedges	1	1
Garlic cloves, minced	2	2
(or 1/2 tsp., 2 mL, powder)		
Dried crushed chilies	1/2 tsp.	2 mL
Boneless, skinless chicken breast halves,	1 lb.	454 g
thinly sliced (see Tip, page 101)		
Low-sodium prepared chicken broth	3 cups	750 mL
Sweet chili sauce	2 tbsp.	30 mL
Low-sodium soy sauce	1 tbsp.	15 mL
Shredded suey choy (Chinese cabbage)	2 cups	500 mL
Sliced red pepper	1 cup	250 mL
Rice vinegar	1 tbsp.	15 mL
Sesame oil (for flavour)	1/2 tsp.	2 mL
Rice vermicelli	8 oz.	225 g
Boiling water		

Put mushrooms into small bowl. Pour boiling water over top until covered. Let stand for about 20 minutes until softened. Drain. Remove and discard stems. Thinly slice. Set aside.

Stir water into cornstarch in small cup until smooth. Set aside.

Heat cooking oil in large pot or Dutch oven on medium. Add next 3 ingredients. Cook for about 5 minutes, stirring often, until onion is tender-crisp.

Add chicken. Cook for 5 to 10 minutes, stirring occasionally, until chicken is no longer pink inside.

Add next 3 ingredients. Stir. Cover. Cook for about 5 minutes, stirring occasionally, until boiling.

Add next 4 ingredients. Stir. Cover. Cook for about 2 minutes until cabbage and red pepper are tender-crisp. Stir cornstarch mixture. Add to chicken mixture. Add mushrooms. Heat and stir for about 1 minute until sauce is boiling and slightly thickened.

(continued on next page)

Put vermicelli into large bowl. Pour boiling water over top until covered. Cover. Let stand for about 5 minutes until vermicelli is tender. Drain. Spoon into 4 bowls. Spoon chicken mixture onto vermicelli. Serves 4.

1 serving: 465 Calories; 5.8 g Total Fat (2.1 g Mono, 1.5 g Poly, 0.8 g Sat); 66 mg Cholesterol; 69 g Carbohydrate; 4 g Fibre; 34 g Protein; 732 mg Sodium

Barley Beef Stew

Beef and barley are always good in soup. Now try them together with some colourful veggies in this tasty stew.

Cooking oil	1 tbsp.	15 mL
Stewing beef	1 1/2 lbs.	680 g
Low-sodium prepared beef broth	3 cups	750 mL
Chopped onion	1 cup	250 mL
Fennel bulb (white part only), thinly sliced	1	1
Sliced red pepper	2 cups	500 mL
Pearl barley	1/2 cup	125 mL
Chopped fresh oregano	1 tbsp.	15 mL
(or 3/4 tsp., 4 mL, dried)		
Pepper	1/4 tsp.	1 mL
Fresh spinach, stems removed, lightly packed	2 cups	500 mL

Heat cooking oil in large pot or Dutch oven on medium. Add beef. Cook for about 10 minutes, stirring occasionally, until browned.

Add next 3 ingredients. Stir. Bring to a boil. Reduce heat to medium-low. Cover. Simmer for about 1 1/2 hours, stirring occasionally, until beef is tender.

Add next 4 ingredients. Stir. Cover. Simmer for about 45 minutes, stirring occasionally, until barley is tender.

Add spinach. Heat and stir for about 1 minute until spinach is wilted. Serves 6.

1 serving: 323 Calories; 12.6 g Total Fat (5.6 g Mono, 1.3 g Poly, 4.2 g Sat); 63 mg Cholesterol; 24 g Carbohydrate; 3 g Fibre; 29 g Protein; 444 mg Sodium

Pictured on page 90.

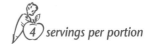

Beef and Eggplant Stew

Deep colour and rich flavour make this stew a real winner for dinner! Serve with buns or ciabatta bread.

Olive (or cooking) oil	2 tsp.	10 mL
Stewing beef	1 lb.	454 g
Olive (or cooking) oil	2 tsp.	10 mL
Cubed eggplant	4 cups	1 L
Chopped onion	1 1/2 cups	375 mL
Can of diced tomatoes (with juice)	14 oz.	398 mL
Dry (or alcohol-free) red wine	3/4 cup	175 mL
Tomato paste (see Tip, page 87)	1/4 cup	60 mL
Can of artichoke hearts, drained and quartered	14 oz.	398 mL
Kalamata olives	1/4 cup	60 mL
Chopped fresh mint leaves (or 1 1/2 tsp., 7 mL, dried)	2 tbsp.	30 mL

Heat first amount of olive oil in large pot or Dutch oven on medium-high. Add beef. Cook for 10 to 15 minutes, stirring occasionally, until browned. Transfer to large bowl. Cover to keep warm.

Add second amount of olive oil to same large pot. Reduce heat to medium. Add eggplant and onion. Cook for 5 to 10 minutes, stirring often, until onion is softened.

Add next 3 ingredients. Stir. Bring to a boil. Add beef. Stir. Reduce heat to medium-low. Cover. Simmer for about 1 1/2 hours, stirring occasionally, until beef is very tender. Remove cover. Bring to a boil on medium. Boil gently for about 10 minutes, stirring occasionally, until sauce is thickened.

Add remaining 3 ingredients. Stir. Cook for 3 to 5 minutes, stirring occasionally, until heated through. Serves 4.

1 serving: 382 Calories; 15.7 g Total Fat (8.1 g Mono, 1.1 g Poly, 4.8 g Sat); 63 mg Cholesterol; 26 g Carbohydrate; 7 g Fibre; 30 g Protein; 474 mg Sodium

Beef, Broccoli and Apple Stir-Fry

Beef and broccoli with a sweet apple twist. Perfect with coconut rice.

GINGER MARINADE

Dry sherry	3 tbsp.	50 mL
Low-sodium soy sauce	3 tbsp.	50 mL
Granulated sugar	1 tbsp.	15 mL
Finely grated ginger root (or 1/4 tsp., 1 mL, ground)	1 tsp.	5 mL
Beef rib-eye steak, sliced thinly (see Tip, below)	1/2 lb.	225 g
Cooking oil	1 tsp.	5 mL
Cooking oil	1 tsp.	10 mL
Broccoli florets	2 cups	500 mL
Peeled tart medium cooking apple (such as Granny Smith), thinly sliced	1	1
Green onions, cut into 1 inch (2.5 cm) pieces	4	4

Ginger Marinade: Combine first 4 ingredients in medium bowl. Makes about 1/2 cup (125 mL) marinade. Add beef. Stir until coated. Marinate in refrigerator for 30 minutes, stirring occasionally.

Heat wok or large frying pan on medium-high until very hot. Add first amount of cooking oil. Add beef with marinade. Stir-fry for about 3 minutes until beef is browned. Transfer to separate medium bowl.

Add second amount of cooking oil to same wok. Add remaining 3 ingredients. Stir-fry for about 3 minutes until broccoli is tender-crisp. Add beef mixture. Stir-fry for about 1 minute until heated through. Serves 2.

1 serving: 420 Calories; 23.4 g Total Fat (10.7 g Mono, 2.2 g Poly, 7.9 g Sat); 60 mg Cholesterol; 24 g Carbohydrate; 4 g Fibre; 27 g Protein; 823 mg Sodium

Pictured on page 107.

 To slice meat easily, freeze for about 30 minutes. If using frozen, partially thaw before slicing.

Cashew Vegetable Stir-Fry

An appealing mix of tender-crisp vegetables and crunchy cashews. Ginger and hoisin flavours linger delightfully on the palate. Serve with thick Shanghai noodles or steamed jasmine rice.

Water	1 tbsp.	15 mL
Cornstarch	2 tsp.	10 mL
Chinese dried mushrooms	12	12
Boiling water		
Cooking oil	2 tsp.	10 mL
Large onion, cut into thin wedges	1	1
Fresh chili pepper, finely chopped	1	1
(see Tip, page 117)		
Garlic cloves, minced	2	2
(or 1/2 tsp., 2 mL, powder)		
Finely grated ginger root	1/2 tsp.	2 mL
(or 1/8 tsp., 0.5 mL, ground)		
Snow peas, trimmed	2 cups	500 mL
Medium red peppers, cut into thin strips	2	2
Green onions, cut into 1 inch	12	12
(2.5 cm) pieces		
Medium carrot, cut julienne (see Note)	1	1
Oyster sauce	2 tbsp.	30 mL
Hoisin sauce	2 tbsp.	30 mL
Liquid honey	1 tbsp.	15 mL
Finely shredded fresh basil	2 tbsp.	30 mL
Raw cashews, toasted (see Tip, page 47)	1/3 cup	75 mL

Stir water into cornstarch in small cup until smooth. Set aside.

Put mushrooms into small bowl. Pour boiling water over top until covered. Let stand for about 20 minutes until softened. Drain. Remove and discard stems. Thinly slice. Set aside.

Heat wok or large frying pan on medium-high until very hot. Add cooking oil. Add next 4 ingredients. Stir-fry for about 2 minutes until fragrant.

Add next 4 ingredients. Stir-fry for 2 minutes.

Combine next 3 ingredients in separate small cup. Add to snow pea mixture. Add mushrooms. Stir-fry for 2 to 3 minutes until vegetables are tender-crisp. Stir cornstarch mixture. Add to vegetables. Stir-fry for about 1 minute until sauce is boiling and thickened.

Add basil and cashews. Stir-fry for about 1 minute until heated through. Serves 6.

(continued on next page)

1 serving: 176 Calories; 5.8 g Total Fat (3.2 g Mono, 1.3 g Poly, 0.9 g Sat); 0 mg Cholesterol; 29 g Carbohydrate; 4 g Fibre; 5 g Protein; 572 mg Sodium

Pictured on page 108.

Note: To julienne vegetables, cut into 1/8 inch (3 mm) strips that resemble matchsticks.

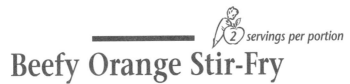 *servings per portion*

Beefy Orange Stir-Fry

Sweet citrus and tender-crisp snow peas make this beefy dish hard to resist.
Serve with brown rice for a complete meal.

Water	1 tbsp.	15 mL
Cornstarch	2 tsp.	10 mL
Black bean sauce (pourable)	2 tbsp.	30 mL
Liquid honey	1 tbsp.	15 mL
Sesame oil (optional)	1/2 tsp.	2 mL
Cooking oil	2 tsp.	10 mL
Beef top sirloin steak, thinly sliced (see Tip, page 101)	1/2 lb.	225 g
Snow peas, trimmed	2 cups	500 mL
Medium oranges, segmented	4	4
Sesame seeds, toasted (see Tip, page 47)	2 tsp.	10 mL

Stir water into cornstarch in small cup until smooth. Add next 3 ingredients. Stir. Set aside.

Heat wok or large frying pan on medium-high until very hot. Add cooking oil. Add beef. Stir-fry for about 2 minutes until beef starts to brown.

Add snow peas. Stir-fry for about 2 minutes until peas are tender-crisp.

Stir cornstarch mixture. Add to beef mixture. Add orange segments. Stir gently until heated through and sauce is slightly thickened. Remove to large serving dish.

Sprinkle with sesame seeds. Serves 4.

1 serving: 248 Calories; 9 g Total Fat (4.2 g Mono, 1.5 g Poly, 2.4 g Sat); 28 mg Cholesterol; 29 g Carbohydrate; 4 g Fibre; 15 g Protein; 345 mg Sodium

Pictured on page 108.

Choy Sum Pork Stir-Fry

A tasty mixture of pork and greens seasoned with a pungent marinade.

FIVE-SPICE MARINADE

Low-sodium soy sauce	2 tbsp.	30 mL
Garlic cloves, minced	3	3
(or 3/4 tsp., 4 mL, powder)		
Finely grated ginger root	2 tsp.	10 mL
(or 1/2 tsp., 2 mL, ground)		
Granulated sugar	2 tsp.	10 mL
Chinese five-spice powder	1/4 tsp.	1 mL
Pork tenderloin, trimmed of fat and thinly sliced (see Tip, page 101)	1/2 lb.	225 g
Cooking oil	1 tsp.	5 mL
Coarsely chopped choy sum (or broccoli), stems trimmed 1 inch (2.5 cm) from end	4 cups	1 L
Sugar snap peas, trimmed	1 cup	250 mL
Green onions, cut into 2 inch (5 cm) pieces	12	12
Sesame seeds, toasted (see Tip, page 47)	1 tsp.	5 mL

Five-Spice Marinade: Combine first 5 ingredients in small bowl. Makes about 2 tbsp. (30 mL) marinade.

Put pork into medium resealable freezer bag. Add marinade. Seal bag. Turn until coated. Marinate in refrigerator for 1 hour, turning occasionally.

Heat wok or large frying pan on medium-high until very hot. Add cooking oil. Add pork with marinade. Stir-fry for 3 minutes.

Add next 3 ingredients. Stir-fry for 3 to 5 minutes until vegetables are tender-crisp. Remove to medium serving dish.

Sprinkle with sesame seeds. Serves 4.

1 serving: 134 Calories; 4.2 g Total Fat (1.9 g Mono, 0.9 g Poly, 1 g Sat); 35 mg Cholesterol; 10 g Carbohydrate; 2 g Fibre; 15 g Protein; 327 mg Sodium

Chicken Pineapple Noodles

Sweet 'n' sour and just a little spicy!

Medium rice stick noodles	4 1/2 oz.	125 g
Boiling water		
Cooking oil	1 tbsp.	15 mL
Boneless, skinless chicken breast halves,	1 lb.	454 g
thinly sliced (see Tip, page 101)		
Garlic cloves, minced	2	2
(or 1/2 tsp., 2 mL, powder)		
Dried crushed chilies	1/2 tsp.	2 mL
Fresh (or frozen, thawed) green beans,	2 1/4 cups	550 mL
cut into 1 1/2 inch (3.8 cm) pieces		
Thinly sliced red pepper	1 1/2 cups	375 mL
Can of pineapple tidbits, drained	14 oz.	398 mL
Lime juice	1/4 cup	60 mL
Chopped fresh cilantro or parsley	3 tbsp.	50 mL
Low-sodium soy sauce	2 tbsp.	30 mL
Liquid honey	2 tbsp.	30 mL
Fish sauce	1 tsp.	5 mL
Coarsely chopped unsalted peanuts,	2 tbsp.	30 mL
toasted (see Tip, page 47)		

Put noodles into large bowl. Pour boiling water over top until covered. Let stand for 10 to 15 minutes until softened. Drain. Set aside.

Heat wok or large frying pan on medium-high until very hot. Add cooking oil. Add next 3 ingredients. Stir-fry for about 3 minutes until chicken starts to brown.

Add green beans and red pepper. Stir-fry for about 3 minutes until vegetables are tender-crisp.

Add noodles and next 6 ingredients. Stir-fry for about 1 minute until heated through. Remove to large serving dish.

Sprinkle with peanuts. Serves 4.

1 serving: 415 Calories; 8.3 g Total Fat (3.7 g Mono, 2.3 g Poly, 1.1 g Sat); 66 mg Cholesterol; 55 g Carbohydrate; 4 g Fibre; 32 g Protein; 347 mg Sodium

Shrimp and Pea Stir-Fry

A colourful combination in a light, minty sauce. Serve over rice.

Cooking oil	2 tsp.	10 mL
Small onion, cut into thin wedges	1	1
Sugar snap peas, trimmed	2 cups	500 mL
Julienned carrot (see Note)	1 cup	250 mL
Uncooked medium shrimp (peeled and deveined)	1 lb.	454 g
Chopped fresh mint leaves	3 tbsp.	50 mL
Sweet chili sauce	3 tbsp.	50 mL
Lime juice	1 tbsp.	15 mL

Heat wok or large frying pan on medium-high until very hot. Add cooking oil. Add onion. Stir-fry for about 2 minutes until onion starts to brown.

Add sugar snap peas and carrots. Stir-fry for about 2 minutes until peas are tender-crisp.

Add remaining 4 ingredients. Stir-fry for 3 to 5 minutes until shrimp turn pink and carrots are tender-crisp. Serves 4.

1 serving: 176 Calories; 4.1 g Total Fat (1.6 g Mono, 1.4 g Poly, 0.5 g Sat); 129 mg Cholesterol; 15 g Carbohydrate; 3 g Fibre; 20 g Protein; 314 mg Sodium

Pictured on page 108.

Note: To julienne vegetables, cut into 1/8 inch (3 mm) strips that resemble matchsticks.

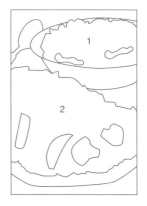

1. Chicken Vegetable Fried Rice, page 111
2. Beef, Broccoli and Apple Stir-Fry, page 101

Props courtesy of: Out of the Fire Studio

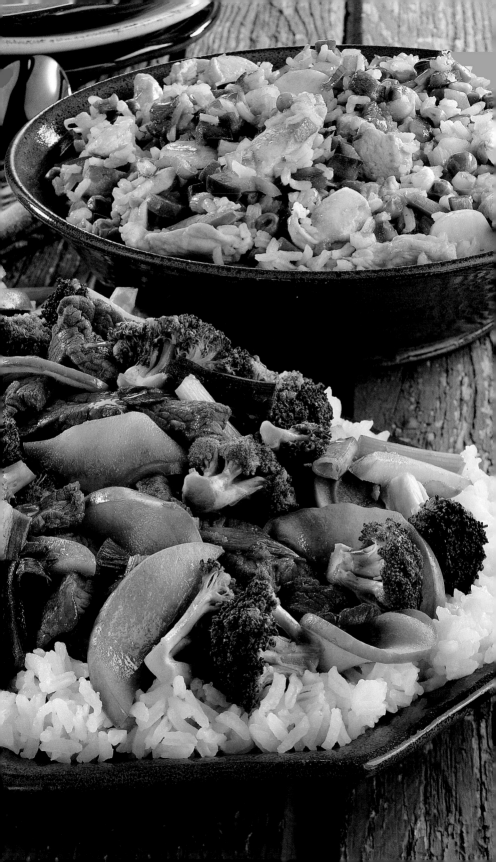

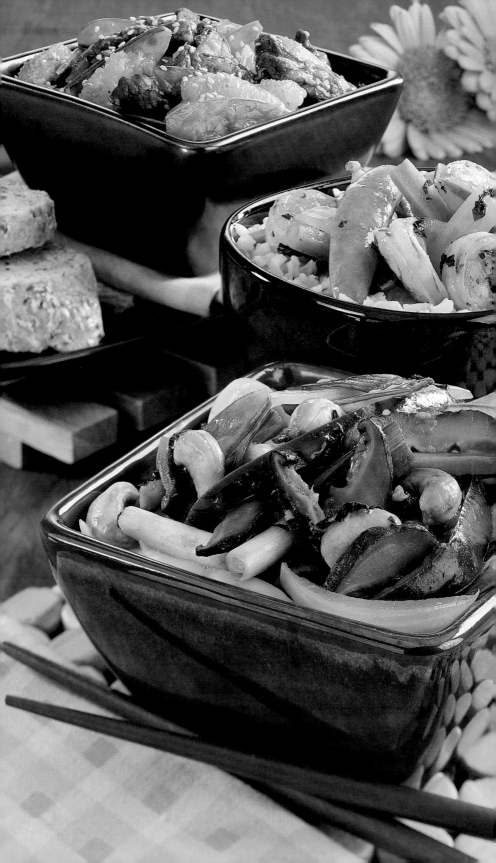

Chicken Zucchini Stir-Fry

Refreshing lemon and dill add a lively splash and dash of flavour to tender chicken and mild zucchini. Very tasty!

Cooking oil	2 tsp.	10 mL
Boneless, skinless chicken breast halves, thinly sliced (see Tip, page 101)	1 lb.	454 g
Medium zucchini (with peel), cut julienne (see Note)	1	1
Frozen peas	2/3 cup	150 mL
Lemon juice	1 tbsp.	15 mL
Chopped fresh dill (or 1/2 tsp., 2 mL, dried)	2 tsp.	10 mL
Garlic cloves, minced (or 1/2 tsp., 2 mL, powder)	2	2
Pepper	1/8 tsp.	0.5 mL

Heat wok or large frying pan on medium-high until very hot. Add cooking oil. Add chicken. Stir-fry for about 3 minutes until chicken starts to brown.

Add remaining 6 ingredients. Stir-fry for about 5 minutes until chicken is no longer pink inside and zucchini is tender-crisp. Serves 4.

1 serving: 175 Calories; 4.4 g Total Fat (1.8 g Mono, 1.2 g Poly, 0.7 g Sat); 66 mg Cholesterol; 6 g Carbohydrate; 2 g Fibre; 27 g Protein; 30 mg Sodium

Note: To julienne vegetables, cut into 1/8 inch (3 mm) strips that resemble matchsticks.

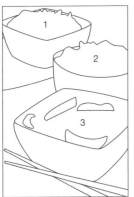

1. Beefy Orange Stir-Fry, page 103
2. Shrimp and Pea Stir-Fry, page 106
3. Cashew Vegetable Stir-Fry, page 102

Props courtesy of: Cherison Enterprises Inc.
Danesco Inc.

Mushroom Noodle Stir-Fry

An interesting fusion of flavours in a light, creamy sauce. Definitely for mushroom lovers!

Milk	1/2 cup	125 mL
Cornstarch	2 tsp.	10 mL
Fresh thin Chinese-style egg noodles	5 1/4 oz.	150 g
Boiling water	2 cups	500 mL
Cooking oil	1 tbsp.	15 mL
Sliced fresh brown (or white) mushrooms	4 cups	1 L
Garlic cloves, minced	2	2
(or 1/2 tsp., 2 mL, powder)		
Frozen peas	1 cup	250 mL
Prepared vegetable (or low-sodium	1/2 cup	125 mL
chicken) broth		
Pepper	1/4 tsp.	1 mL
Grated Parmesan cheese	1/3 cup	75 mL
Chopped fresh parsley	3 tbsp.	50 mL
(or 2 1/4 tsp., 11 mL, flakes)		

Stir milk into cornstarch in small cup until smooth. Set aside.

Cook noodles in boiling water in large uncovered saucepan for 1 minute. Stir to loosen noodles. Drain. Return to same saucepan. Cover to keep warm.

Heat wok or large frying pan on medium-high until very hot. Add cooking oil. Add mushrooms and garlic. Stir-fry for about 4 minutes until mushrooms start to brown.

Add next 3 ingredients. Stir-fry for 1 minute. Stir cornstarch mixture. Add to mushroom mixture. Stir-fry for about 1 minute until sauce is boiling and thickened. Add noodles. Stir-fry for about 1 minute until heated through.

Add Parmesan cheese and parsley. Toss well. Serves 4.

1 serving: 193 Calories; 7.5 g Total Fat (3.1 g Mono, 1.5 g Poly, 2.4 g Sat); 21 mg Cholesterol; 22 g Carbohydrate; 4 g Fibre; 11 g Protein; 333 mg Sodium

Chicken Vegetable Fried Rice

A colourful blend with delicious smoky flavour. A meal all by itself!

Cooking oil	1 tbsp.	15 mL
Boneless, skinless chicken breast halves, thinly sliced (see Tip, page 101)	12 oz.	340 g
Chopped green pepper	1 cup	250 mL
Chopped red pepper	1 cup	250 mL
Frozen peas	1 cup	250 mL
Can of sliced water chestnuts, drained	8 oz.	227 mL
Thinly sliced green onion	1/2 cup	125 mL
Chopped low-fat deli ham	1/2 cup	125 mL
Low-sodium soy sauce	1 1/2 tbsp.	25 mL
Hoisin sauce	1 tbsp.	15 mL
Sweet chili sauce	1 tbsp.	15 mL
Cold cooked long-grain white rice (about 2/3 cup, 150 mL, uncooked)	2 cups	500 mL

Heat wok or large frying pan on medium-high until very hot. Add cooking oil. Add chicken. Stir-fry for 3 to 5 minutes until chicken is no longer pink inside.

Add next 6 ingredients. Stir-fry for 2 to 3 minutes until peppers are tender-crisp.

Combine next 3 ingredients in small cup. Add to chicken mixture. Stir.

Add rice. Stir-fry for about 5 minutes until heated through and liquid is almost evaporated. Serves 6.

1 serving: 272 Calories; 5.2 g Total Fat (2.4 g Mono, 1.2 g Poly, 1 g Sat); 41 mg Cholesterol; 36 g Carbohydrate; 3 g Fibre; 20 g Protein; 448 mg Sodium

Pictured on page 107.

Pictured on page 107.

Paré Pointer

"Where were you when the lights went out?" "In the dark!"

Pork and Apple Stir-Fry

A delicious combination that's ready in just minutes. Serve over spaetzle, egg noodles or oven-roasted potatoes.

Water	1 tbsp.	15 mL
Cornstarch	1 tbsp.	15 mL
Apple juice	1/3 cup	75 mL
Low-sodium soy sauce	1 tbsp.	15 mL
Liquid honey	1 tbsp.	15 mL
Pepper	1/8 tsp.	0.5 mL
Cooking oil	1 tbsp.	15 mL
Pork tenderloin, trimmed of fat and thinly sliced (see Tip, page 101)	3/4 lb.	340 g
Chopped cabbage	2 1/2 cups	625 mL
Peeled medium cooking apples (such as McIntosh), sliced	2	2
Chopped pecans, toasted (see Tip, page 47)	1/3 cup	75 mL

Stir water into cornstarch in small bowl until smooth. Add next 4 ingredients. Stir.

Heat wok or large frying pan on medium-high until very hot. Add cooking oil. Add pork. Stir-fry for 2 to 3 minutes until pork starts to brown.

Add cabbage and apple. Stir-fry for about 2 minutes until cabbage just starts to soften. Stir cornstarch mixture. Add to pork mixture. Stir-fry for about 1 minute until sauce is boiling and thickened.

Add pecans. Stir well. Serves 4.

1 serving: 292 Calories; 15.2 g Total Fat (8.4 g Mono, 3.3 g Poly, 2.4 g Sat); 47 mg Cholesterol; 20 g Carbohydrate; 2 g Fibre; 20 g Protein; 170 mg Sodium

Sweet Tofu and Vegetables

A sweet and spicy combination that's great served with noodles.

Low-sodium soy sauce	1 tbsp.	15 mL
Liquid honey	1 tbsp.	15 mL
Dry sherry	1 tbsp.	15 mL
Cornstarch	2 tsp.	10 mL
Chili paste (sambal oelek)	1 tsp.	5 mL
Package of extra-firm tofu, drained, cut into 1/2 inch (1.2 cm) cubes	12 1/4 oz.	350 g
Peanut (or cooking) oil	1 tbsp.	15 mL
Snow peas, trimmed	2 cups	500 mL
Coarsely chopped suey choy (Chinese cabbage)	2 cups	500 mL
Thinly sliced green pepper	1 cup	250 mL
Green onions, cut into 1 inch (2.5 cm) pieces	4	4
Garlic clove, minced (or 1/4 tsp., 1 mL, powder)	1	1

Combine first 5 ingredients in medium bowl. Add tofu. Stir gently.

Heat wok or large frying pan on medium-high until very hot. Add peanut oil. Add remaining 5 ingredients. Stir-fry for 1 minute. Add tofu mixture. Stir gently for 3 to 4 minutes until sauce is boiling and thickened and vegetables are tender-crisp. Serves 4.

1 serving: 235 Calories; 11.4 g Total Fat (3.3 g Mono, 5.6 g Poly, 1.7 g Sat); 0 mg Cholesterol; 20 g Carbohydrate; 3 g Fibre; 17 g Protein; 144 mg Sodium

 tip To maintain the nutrients in your fresh vegetables, steam or cook them with as little water as possible. Use the nutrient-rich cooking water in your gravies and sauces.

Pork and Spinach Stir-Fry

A fragrant stir-fry that's made for pasta!

Cooking oil	1 tbsp.	15 mL
Boneless pork loin chops, trimmed of fat and thinly sliced (see Tip, page 101)	3/4 lb.	340 g
Fresh asparagus, trimmed of tough ends and cut into 1 inch (2.5 cm) pieces	1/2 lb.	225 g
Lemon juice	1 tbsp.	15 mL
Garlic cloves, minced (or 1/2 tsp., 2 mL, powder)	2	2
Chili paste (sambal oelek)	1/2 tsp.	2 mL
Pepper	1/8 tsp.	0.5 mL
Fresh spinach, stems removed, lightly packed	3 cups	750 mL
Finely shredded fresh basil	2 tbsp.	30 mL
Grated Parmesan cheese	2 tbsp.	30 mL

Heat wok or large frying pan on medium-high until very hot. Add cooking oil. Add pork. Stir-fry for 2 minutes.

Add next 5 ingredients. Stir-fry for about 2 minutes until asparagus is tender-crisp.

Add spinach and basil. Stir-fry for about 1 minute until spinach is just wilted. Remove to medium serving dish.

Sprinkle with Parmesan cheese. Serves 4.

1 serving: 227 Calories; 13.9 g Total Fat (6.4 g Mono, 2.2 g Poly, 4.1 g Sat); 52 mg Cholesterol; 5 g Carbohydrate; 2 g Fibre; 21 g Protein; 132 mg Sodium

Paré Pointer

A chicken's favourite dessert is coop-cakes.

Tomato Fennel Risotto

Fennel, lemon and dill are refreshing additions to this creamy dish. Fabulous with fish.

Low-sodium prepared chicken (or vegetable) broth	3 cups	750 mL
Cooking oil	2 tsp.	10 mL
Fennel bulb (white part only), thinly sliced	1	1
Finely chopped onion	3/4 cup	175 mL
Arborio (or other short-grain white) rice	1 cup	250 mL
Dry (or alcohol-free) white wine	1/4 cup	60 mL
Medium tomatoes, peeled (see Tip, page 38) and chopped	2	2
Medium zucchini (with peel), diced	1/2	1/2
Chopped fresh dill (or 3/4 tsp., 4 mL, dried)	1 tbsp.	15 mL
Lemon juice	2 tsp.	10 mL
Pepper	1/8 tsp.	0.5 mL

Bring broth to a boil in medium saucepan on medium-high. Reduce heat to low. Cover to keep warm.

Heat cooking oil in large saucepan on medium. Add fennel and onion. Cook for about 7 minutes, stirring occasionally, until fennel is softened.

Add rice. Stir. Add wine. Heat and stir for about 1 minute until wine is almost absorbed.

Add tomato and 1 cup (250 mL) warm broth. Heat and stir for about 6 minutes until broth is almost absorbed. Add 1 cup (250 mL) warm broth. Heat and stir for 8 to 10 minutes until broth is almost absorbed.

Add zucchini and remaining broth. Heat and stir for about 10 minutes until broth is almost absorbed and zucchini is tender-crisp.

Add remaining 3 ingredients. Stir well. Serves 6.

1 serving: 175 Calories; 1.9 g Total Fat (1 g Mono, 0.6 g Poly, 0.2 g Sat); 0 mg Cholesterol; 33 g Carbohydrate; 1 g Fibre; 5 g Protein; 331 mg Sodium

Marinated Mushrooms

Always good! These tender mushrooms with a chili pepper bite are perfect with pasta or roasted meats. Add another chili for more heat.

Fresh chili peppers (with seeds), chopped (see Tip, page 117)	2	2
Cooking oil	1 cup	250 mL
White wine vinegar	1/3 cup	75 mL
Granulated sugar	1 tbsp.	15 mL
Garlic cloves, minced (or 3/4 tsp., 4 mL, powder)	3	3
Salt	1 tsp.	5 mL
Pepper	1/2 tsp.	2 mL
Small fresh white mushrooms	1 1/2 lbs.	680 g
Diced red pepper	1 cup	250 mL

Combine first 7 ingredients in large saucepan. Heat and stir on medium for about 5 minutes until boiling and sugar is dissolved.

Add mushrooms. Cook for about 5 minutes, stirring often, until mushrooms are softened.

Add red pepper. Cook for 3 to 5 minutes, stirring occasionally, until red pepper is tender-crisp. Drain. Serves 8.

1 serving: 163 Calories; 14.8 g Total Fat (8.5 g Mono, 4.4 g Poly, 1.1 g Sat); 0 mg Cholesterol; 8 g Carbohydrate; 2 g Fibre; 2 g Protein; 153 mg Sodium

Potato Pan Cake

Shredded potato and onion baked in a pan and cut like a cake. Almost too easy.

Cold water		
Potatoes, peeled	2 lbs.	900 g
Large eggs	2	2
Finely chopped onion	1/2 cup	125 mL
Garlic and herb no-salt seasoning (such as Mrs. Dash)	1/2 tsp.	2 mL
Pepper	1/4 tsp.	1 mL
Hot milk	1 cup	250 mL

(continued on next page)

Side Dishes

Pour cold water into large bowl until about half full. Grate potatoes into water (to prevent browning), adding more water if necessary to keep covered.

Combine next 4 ingredients in separate large bowl. Drain potato. Squeeze to remove excess water. Add to egg mixture. Stir well.

Slowly add hot milk, stirring constantly until potato is coated. Spread evenly in greased 9 x 9 inch (22 x 22 cm) pan. Bake, uncovered, in 375°F (190°C) oven for about 1 hour until golden. Let stand for 5 minutes before cutting. Cuts into 9 pieces.

1 piece: 82 Calories; 1.5 g Total Fat (0.5 g Mono, 0.2 g Poly, 0.6 g Sat); 49 mg Cholesterol; 14 g Carbohydrate; 1 g Fibre; 4 g Protein; 32 mg Sodium

Stir-Fried Honey Greens

Tender-crisp vegetables glisten with a gently sweet honey sauce.

Hoisin sauce	1 tbsp.	15 mL
Liquid honey	1 tbsp.	15 mL
Cornstarch	2 tsp.	10 mL
Cooking oil	1 tsp.	5 mL
Chopped bok choy	3 cups	750 mL
Fresh asparagus, trimmed of tough ends and cut into 2 inch (5 cm) pieces	1 lb.	454 g

Combine first 3 ingredients in small cup.

Heat wok or large frying pan on medium-high until very hot. Add cooking oil. Add bok choy and asparagus. Stir-fry for 4 to 5 minutes until vegetables are tender-crisp. Stir cornstarch mixture. Add to vegetable mixture. Stir-fry for about 1 minute until sauce is boiling and thickened. Serves 6.

1 serving: 48 Calories; 1 g Total Fat (0.5 g Mono, 0.3 g Poly, 0.1 g Sat); 0 mg Cholesterol; 9 g Carbohydrate; 1 g Fibre; 2 g Protein; 91 mg Sodium

 tip
Hot peppers contain capsaicin in the seeds and ribs. Removing the seeds and ribs will reduce the heat. Wear rubber gloves when handling peppers and avoid touching your eyes. Wash your hands well afterwards.

Two-Potato Scallop

One potato, two potato—there's a treat for you in store. Taste it once, it's very nice, and then come have some more!

Hard margarine (or butter)	1/4 cup	60 mL
All-purpose flour	2 tbsp.	30 mL
Milk	2 cups	500 mL
Grated Parmesan cheese	3 tbsp.	50 mL
Ground thyme	1/4 tsp.	1 mL
Pepper (white is best)	1/4 tsp.	1 mL
Potatoes, peeled and very thinly sliced	1 lb.	454 g
Peeled fresh orange-fleshed sweet potatoes, very thinly sliced	1 lb.	454 g
Chopped onion	1/2 cup	125 mL

Melt margarine in medium saucepan on medium. Add flour. Heat and stir for 1 minute.

Slowly add next 4 ingredients, stirring constantly. Heat and stir for about 7 minutes until boiling and thickened.

Layer half of potato, half of sweet potato and half of onion, in order given, in greased 2 quart (2 L) casserole. Pour half of milk mixture evenly over top. Repeat with remaining potato, sweet potato, onion and milk mixture. Bake in 375°F (190°C) oven for about 1 hour until potatoes are tender. Serves 6.

1 serving: 261 Calories; 10.3 g Total Fat (5.8 g Mono, 1 g Poly, 2.9 g Sat); 6 mg Cholesterol; 36 g Carbohydrate; 3 g Fibre; 7 g Protein; 210 mg Sodium

Dilled Zucchini

Tender-crisp zucchini accented with orange and dill. A palette of green that needs to be seen!

Hard margarine (or butter)	2 tsp.	10 mL
Medium zucchini (with peel), cut julienne (see Note)	3	3
Orange juice	2 tbsp.	30 mL
Cornstarch	1 tsp.	5 mL
Chopped fresh dill (or 3/4 tsp., 4 mL, dried)	1 tbsp.	15 mL
Pepper, sprinkle		

(continued on next page)

Melt margarine in medium frying pan on medium-high. Add zucchini. Cook for about 3 minutes, stirring often, until tender-crisp.

Stir orange juice into cornstarch in small cup until smooth. Add to zucchini mixture, stirring constantly. Heat and stir until boiling and thickened.

Add dill and pepper. Heat and stir for another minute. Serves 4.

1 serving: 38 Calories; 2.1 g Total Fat (1.3 g Mono, 0.3 g Poly, 0.4 g Sat); 0 mg Cholesterol; 4 g Carbohydrate; 2 g Fibre; 1 g Protein; 26 mg Sodium

Note: To julienne vegetables, cut into 1/8 inch (3 mm) strips that resemble matchsticks.

Marinated Celery

Crisp celery marinated in a tangy vinaigrette makes a tasty addition to a barbecue meal.

Celery ribs, cut diagonally into 1/2 inch (12 mm) pieces	2 lbs.	900 g
Water		
Cooking oil	1/3 cup	75 mL
Red wine vinegar	1/3 cup	75 mL
Roasted red peppers, drained, blotted dry, finely chopped	1/4 cup	60 mL
Granulated sugar	2 tbsp.	30 mL
Dry mustard	1 tsp.	5 mL
Dijon mustard	1/2 tsp.	2 mL

Put celery into large pot or Dutch oven. Add water. Cover. Bring to a boil on medium-high. Boil gently for 1 minute. Drain. Rinse with cold water until cold. Drain well.

Combine all 6 ingredients in large bowl. Add celery. Stir until coated. Cover. Chill for 4 hours. Drain. Serves 8.

1 serving: 68 Calories; 4.9 g Total Fat (2.8 g Mono, 1.5 g Poly, 0.4 g Sat); 0 mg Cholesterol; 6 g Carbohydrate; 2 g Fibre; 1 g Protein; 100 mg Sodium

Polynesian Sweet Potatoes

Almost sweet enough to be dessert. Serve with roast beef or pork.

Hard margarine (or butter)	1/2 tsp.	2 mL
Chopped pecans	2 1/2 tbsp.	37 mL
Medium unsweetened coconut	2 tbsp.	30 mL
Unpeeled fresh orange-fleshed sweet potatoes (or yams)	2 1/2 lbs.	1.1 kg
Mashed banana (about 1 medium)	1/3 cup	75 mL
Orange juice	1/4 cup	60 mL
Brown sugar, packed	2 tbsp.	30 mL
Salt	1/2 tsp.	2 mL
Maple (or maple-flavoured) syrup	2 tbsp.	30 mL

Melt margarine in small frying pan on medium. Add pecans. Heat and stir for 1 minute. Add coconut. Heat and stir for 2 to 5 minutes until fragrant and coconut is golden. Set aside.

Randomly poke several holes with fork into each sweet potato. Wrap each with paper towel. Microwave on high (100%) for 18 to 20 minutes, turning potatoes at halftime, until tender. Discard paper towels. Slice each potato in half lengthwise. Scoop flesh into large bowl. Discard skins.

Add next 4 ingredients. Mash well. Spread evenly in ungreased 1 1/2 quart (1.5 L) shallow baking dish. Sprinkle pecan mixture evenly over top. Bake in 325°F (160°C) oven for 15 to 20 minutes until heated through.

Drizzle with syrup. Serves 6.

1 serving: 179 Calories; 4 g Total Fat (1.6 g Mono, 0.7 g Poly, 1.4 g Sat); 0 mg Cholesterol; 35 g Carbohydrate; 3 g Fibre; 2 g Protein; 216 mg Sodium

 Set reasonable goals when changing eating habits in order to improve your health. For example, add one fruit serving to your diet every other day until you are more in line with the recommendations of *Canada's Food Guide.*

Stir-Fried Red Cabbage

Savoury Chinese five-spice powder and tart apple add interest to simple cabbage. Satisfyingly crunchy!

White vinegar	2 tbsp.	30 mL
Water	2 tbsp.	30 mL
Cornstarch	1 tsp.	5 mL
Chinese five-spice powder	1/2 tsp.	2 mL
Cooking oil	1 tbsp.	15 mL
Hard margarine (or butter)	1 tbsp.	15 mL
Shredded red cabbage, lightly packed	6 cups	1.5 L
Unpeeled tart medium cooking apple (such as Granny Smith), grated	1/2	1/2
Apple jelly	3 tbsp.	50 mL

Combine first 4 ingredients in small cup. Set aside.

Heat cooking oil and margarine in wok or large frying pan on medium-high until very hot. Add cabbage. Stir-fry for 5 to 10 minutes until tender-crisp.

Add apple and jelly. Stir-fry for 1 minute. Stir cornstarch mixture. Add to cabbage mixture. Heat and stir for 1 to 2 minutes until sauce is boiling and thickened. Serves 6.

1 serving: 91 Calories; 4.5 g Total Fat (2.6 g Mono, 1 g Poly, 0.6 g Sat); 0 mg Cholesterol; 13 g Carbohydrate; 2 g Fibre; 1 g Protein; 35 mg Sodium

Asparagus in Vinaigrette

Pickled asparagus spears accented with pretty pimiento. A pleasant, summery dish.

Fresh asparagus, trimmed of tough ends	1 lb.	454 g
Boiling water		
Ice water		
PIMIENTO MARINADE		
White vinegar	1/3 cup	75 mL
Jar of sliced pimiento (with liquid)	2 oz.	57 mL
Cooking oil	3 tbsp.	50 mL
Sweet pickle relish	3 tbsp.	50 mL
Salt	1 tsp.	5 mL
Granulated sugar	1 tsp.	5 mL
Cayenne pepper	1/8 tsp.	0.5 mL
Garlic powder	1/8 tsp.	0.5 mL

Partially cook asparagus in boiling water in large saucepan for about 5 minutes until bright green. Drain. Immediately plunge into ice water in large bowl. Let stand for about 10 minutes until cold. Drain. Transfer to ungreased 3 quart (3 L) shallow baking dish.

Pimiento Marinade: Combine all 8 ingredients in small bowl. Makes about 1 cup (250 mL) marinade. Pour over asparagus. Turn asparagus until coated. Cover with plastic wrap. Chill for at least 3 hours. Drain. Serves 4.

1 serving: 90 Calories; 5.5 g Total Fat (3.1 g Mono, 1.7 g Poly, 0.4 g Sat); 0 mg Cholesterol; 10 g Carbohydrate; 2 g Fibre; 2 g Protein; 393 mg Sodium

Red Pepper Brussels Sprouts

Bacon and red pepper add delicious flavour to attractive, crisp Brussels sprouts.

Brussels sprouts	3 cups	750 mL
(about 1 1/2 lbs., 680 g)		
Water		
Bacon slices, diced	4	4
Finely chopped red pepper	1/2 cup	125 mL
Finely chopped onion	1/4 cup	60 mL
Hard margarine (or butter)	2 tbsp.	30 mL
Brown sugar, packed	1 tsp.	5 mL
Lemon pepper	1/2 tsp.	2 mL

(continued on next page)

Side Dishes

Cook Brussels sprouts in water in large saucepan until tender-crisp. Drain. Cover to keep warm.

Cook bacon in medium frying pan on medium until crisp. Transfer with slotted spoon to paper towels to drain. Discard drippings, reserving about 2 tsp. (10 mL) in pan.

Heat reserved drippings. Add red pepper and onion. Cook for 5 to 10 minutes, stirring often, until onion is softened.

Add remaining 3 ingredients. Heat and stir for about 1 minute until margarine is melted. Add Brussels sprouts. Stir gently until coated. Serves 4.

1 serving: 176 Calories; 9.5 g Total Fat (5.3 g Mono, 1.2 g Poly, 2.4 g Sat); 5 mg Cholesterol; 19 g Carbohydrate; 7 g Fibre; 8 g Protein; 284 mg Sodium

Creamy Mashed Sweet Potatoes

Sweet, creamy sweet potato to serve with ham. Delicious!

Fresh peeled orange-fleshed sweet potatoes, cubed	2 lbs.	900 g
Water		
Low-fat plain yogurt	1/4 cup	60 mL
Grated Parmesan cheese	1/4 cup	60 mL
Chopped fresh parsley (or 2 1/4 tsp., 11 mL, flakes)	3 tbsp.	50 mL
Granulated sugar	1 tsp.	5 mL
Ground nutmeg	1/8 tsp.	0.5 mL
Pepper	1/8 tsp.	0.5 mL

Cook sweet potato in water in large saucepan until tender. Drain.

Add remaining 6 ingredients. Mash well. Serves 8.

1 serving: 163 Calories; 1.4 g Total Fat (0.3 g Mono, 0.1 g Poly, 0.8 g Sat); 3 mg Cholesterol; 34 g Carbohydrate; 5 g Fibre; 4 g Protein; 79 mg Sodium

Zucchini Cakes

Golden patties of grated zucchini and onion pleasantly seasoned with Italian herbs.
Serve these instead of hash brown potatoes for brunch.

Large egg	1	1
Grated zucchini (with peel), lightly packed	2 1/2 cups	625 mL
Fine dry bread crumbs	1 1/4 cups	300 mL
Finely chopped onion	1/4 cup	60 mL
Italian no-salt seasoning (such as Mrs. Dash)	1 1/2 tsp.	7 mL
Dry mustard	1/4 tsp.	1 mL
All-purpose flour	1/4 cup	60 mL
Cooking oil	1/4 cup	60 mL

Beat egg with fork in large bowl. Add next 5 ingredients. Stir well. Shape mixture into 8 patties, using 1/4 cup (60 mL) for each.

Dredge both sides of each patty in flour in shallow dish.

Heat 2 tbsp. (30 mL) cooking oil in large frying pan on medium. Add 4 patties. Cook for about 2 minutes per side until golden. Remove to large serving plate. Cover to keep warm. Repeat with remaining cooking oil and patties. Makes 8 zucchini cakes. Serves 4.

1 serving: 340 Calories; 18 g Total Fat (9.8 g Mono, 5.1 g Poly, 1.9 g Sat); 54 mg Cholesterol; 37 g Carbohydrate; 3 g Fibre; 8 g Protein; 492 mg Sodium

1. Poppy Seed Fruit Bowl, page 23
2. Creamy Raspberry Cooler, page 12
3. Fruit-Full Muffins, page 148

Props courtesy of: Cherison Enterprises Inc.
Danesco Inc.
Winners

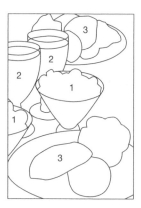

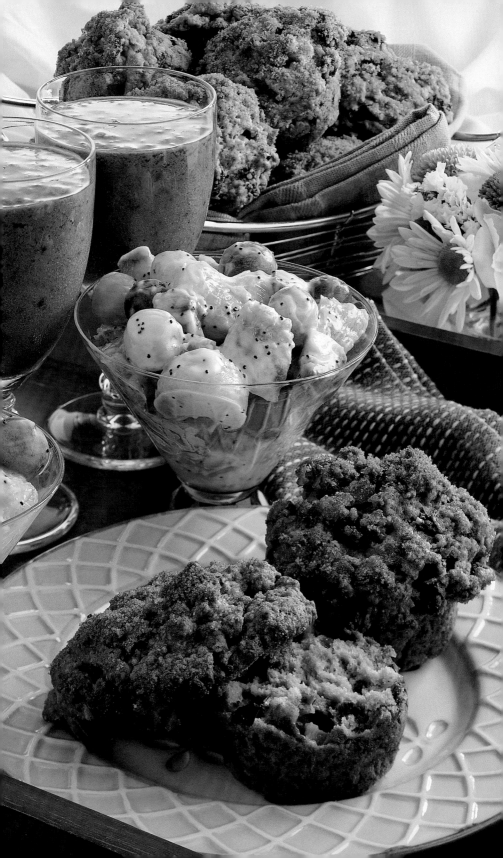

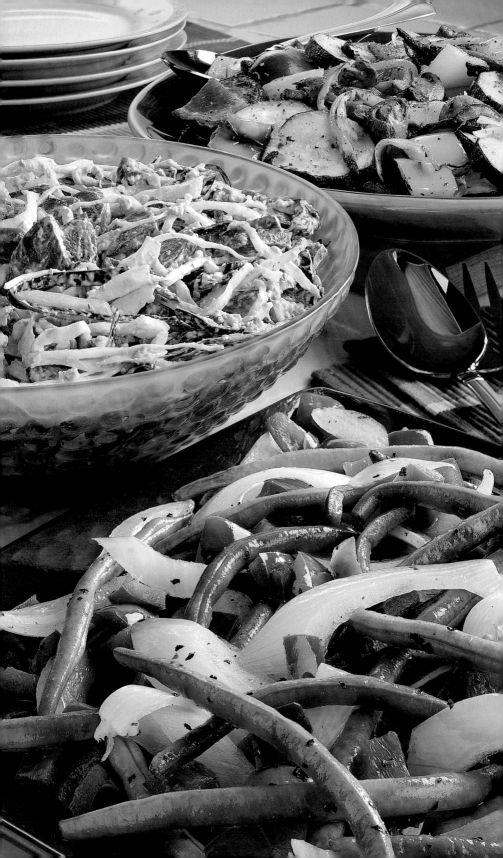

Mediterranean Green Beans

A fragrant, colourful mix that's good any time.

Fresh (or frozen, thawed) green beans	1/2 lb.	225 g
Medium onion, cut into 1/4 inch (6 mm) slices	1	1
Chopped green pepper	1/2 cup	125 mL
Chopped red pepper	1/2 cup	125 mL
Water	1/2 cup	125 mL
Olive (or cooking) oil	2 tbsp.	30 mL
Dried basil	1/2 tsp.	2 mL
Ground cumin	1/4 tsp.	1 mL
Pepper	1/8 tsp.	0.5 mL

Put first 4 ingredients into ungreased 8 x 8 inch (20 x 20 cm) pan.

Combine remaining 5 ingredients in small bowl. Pour over vegetables. Toss until coated. Cover with foil. Bake in 400°F (205°C) oven for 25 to 30 minutes until green beans are tender-crisp. Stir. Drain. Serves 6.

1 serving: 67 Calories; 4.7 g Total Fat (3.4 g Mono, 0.4 g Poly, 0.6 g Sat); 0 mg Cholesterol; 6 g Carbohydrate; 1 g Fibre; 1 g Protein; 4 mg Sodium

Pictured at left.

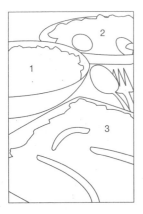

1. Beet Coleslaw, page 22
2. Grilled Mixed Veggies, page 128
3. Mediterranean Green Beans, above

Props courtesy of: Pfaltzgraff Canada

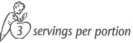

Grilled Mixed Veggies

Combine the goodness of vegetables with smoky barbecue flavour. Delicious!

Medium zucchini (with peel), cut into 1/4 inch (6 mm) slices	3	3
Small red pepper, cut into 1 inch (2.5 cm) pieces	1	1
Small yellow pepper, seeds and ribs removed, cut into 1 inch (2.5 cm) pieces	1	1
Halved fresh white mushrooms	1 cup	250 mL
Sliced red onion	1/2 cup	125 mL
Olive (or cooking) oil	4 tsp.	20 mL
Dried oregano	2 tsp.	10 mL
Lemon juice	1 tsp.	5 mL
No-salt seasoning (such as Mrs. Dash)	1 tsp.	5 mL
Pepper	1/2 tsp.	2 mL

Preheat gas barbecue to medium. Combine all 10 ingredients in large bowl. Transfer to barbecue basket. Place basket on grill. Cook for 25 to 30 minutes, turning basket occasionally, until vegetables are tender-crisp. Serves 4.

1 serving: 91 Calories; 5.1 g Total Fat (3.4 g Mono, 0.6 g Poly, 0.7 g Sat); 0 mg Cholesterol; 11 g Carbohydrate; 4 g Fibre; 3 g Protein; 7 mg Sodium

Pictured on page 126.

Minted Carrots

Carrots need never be boring again!

Water	2/3 cup	150 mL
White vinegar	1/3 cup	75 mL
Granulated sugar	2 tbsp.	30 mL
Coarse ground pepper	1 tsp.	5 mL
Large carrots	3	3
Chopped fresh mint leaves	2 tbsp.	30 mL

(continued on next page)

Combine first 4 ingredients in large bowl.

Peel carrots with vegetable peeler into thin strips. Chop strips. Add to vinegar mixture. Stir until coated. Cover. Chill for at least 3 hours. Drain.

Add mint. Toss. Serves 8.

1 serving: 23 Calories; 0.1 g Total Fat (0 g Mono, 0 g Poly, 0 g Sat); 0 mg Cholesterol; 6 g Carbohydrate; 1 g Fibre; 0 g Protein; 13 mg Sodium

Lemon Butter Fiddleheads

Even though fiddleheads, with their earthy flavour, are only available for a short season each year, they make an interesting and tasty side dish for dinner.

Fresh fiddleheads (see Note)	1 lb.	454 g
Water		
Butter	2 tbsp.	30 mL
Garlic clove, minced	1	1
(or 1/4 tsp., 1 mL, powder)		
Lemon juice	1 tbsp.	15 mL
Maple (or maple-flavoured) syrup	1 tbsp.	15 mL
Grated lemon zest	1/4 tsp.	1 mL
Pepper	1/8 tsp.	0.5 mL

Cook fiddleheads in water in medium saucepan until tender-crisp. Drain.

Melt butter in large frying pan on medium-low. Add garlic. Heat and stir for about 1 minute until fragrant.

Add remaining 4 ingredients. Heat and stir for 1 minute to blend flavours. Add fiddleheads. Stir until coated. Serves 4.

1 serving: 90 Calories; 6.2 g Total Fat (1.7 g Mono, 0.2 g Poly, 3.6 g Sat); 16 mg Cholesterol; 8 g Carbohydrate; 2 g Fibre; 3 g Protein; 62 mg Sodium

Note: To clean fresh fiddleheads, gently rub them between your hands to remove any loose or dry scales. Trim and discard ends. Rinse well.

LEMON BUTTER GREEN BEANS: Omit fiddleheads. Use same amount of fresh green beans.

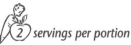

Lentil Rice Pilaf

Warming curry with a hint of sweet honey makes this rice especially nice.

Cooking oil	1 tbsp.	15 mL
Thinly sliced onion	2 cups	500 mL
Chopped red pepper	1 cup	250 mL
Liquid honey	1 tbsp.	15 mL
Curry powder	1 tbsp.	15 mL
Garlic cloves, minced	2	2
(or 1/2 tsp., 2 mL, powder)		
Garlic and herb no-salt seasoning (such as Mrs. Dash)	1/4 tsp.	1 mL
Pepper	1/4 tsp.	1 mL
Low-sodium prepared chicken (or vegetable) broth	2 1/4 cups	550 mL
Can of lentils, rinsed and drained	19 oz.	540 mL
White basmati rice	1 cup	250 mL
Fresh spinach, stems removed, lightly packed	2 cups	500 mL

Heat cooking oil in large pot or Dutch oven on medium. Add onion. Cook for 10 to 15 minutes, stirring often, until caramelized.

Add next 6 ingredients. Stir well.

Add next 3 ingredients. Stir. Bring to a boil. Reduce heat to medium-low. Cover. Simmer for 15 minutes without stirring.

Add spinach. Stir. Cover. Remove from heat. Let stand for 5 to 10 minutes until rice is tender and liquid is absorbed. Serves 4.

1 serving: 374 Calories; 4.7 g Total Fat (2.2 g Mono, 1.4 g Poly, 0.4 g Sat); 0 mg Cholesterol; 71 g Carbohydrate; 7 g Fibre; 14 g Protein; 551 mg Sodium

Paré Pointer

We all like a wishbone but it won't take the place of a backbone.

Strawberries With Orange Custard

A not-too-sweet treat that's fancy enough for company and simple enough for dessert any day.

Icing (confectioner's) sugar	2 tbsp.	30 mL
Orange liqueur (or orange juice)	2 tbsp.	30 mL
Thickly sliced fresh strawberries	6 cups	1.5 L
ORANGE CUSTARD		
Granulated sugar	1/2 cup	125 mL
Cornstarch	1 tbsp.	15 mL
All-purpose flour	1 tbsp.	15 mL
Milk	1 1/2 cups	375 mL
Egg yolks (large)	2	2
Grated orange zest	2 tsp.	10 mL

Combine icing sugar and liqueur in medium bowl. Add strawberries. Stir gently until coated. Cover. Chill for 1 hour.

Orange Custard: Combine first 3 ingredients in medium saucepan. Slowly add milk, stirring constantly until smooth. Heat and stir on medium for about 10 minutes until boiling and thickened. Remove from heat.

Beat egg yolks with fork in small bowl. Add 3 tbsp. (50 mL) hot milk mixture. Stir. Slowly add to hot milk mixture in saucepan, stirring constantly. Heat and stir on medium-low for 2 minutes.

Add orange zest. Stir. Transfer to small bowl. Cover with plastic wrap directly on surface to prevent skin from forming. Chill for about 3 hours until cold. Makes about 1 2/3 cups (400 mL) custard. Spoon strawberry mixture into each of 4 bowls. Spoon custard onto each. Serves 4.

1 serving: 299 Calories; 4.6 g Total Fat (1.4 g Mono, 0.9 g Poly, 1.5 g Sat); 112 mg Cholesterol; 57 g Carbohydrate; 6 g Fibre; 6 g Protein; 55 mg Sodium

KIWI WITH ORANGE CUSTARD: Omit strawberries. Use same amount of sliced kiwifruit.

Fruited Ginger Cake

A gently spiced cake dotted with tasty bits of fruit and nuts. Perfect for tea time.

Orange pekoe tea bag	1	1
Boiling water	1 cup	250 mL
Dark raisins	1 1/2 cups	375 mL
Brown sugar, packed	1 cup	250 mL
Chopped mixed glazed fruit	1/2 cup	125 mL
Large egg	1	1
Applesauce	1/2 cup	125 mL
Chopped walnuts (or almonds)	1/3 cup	75 mL
Minced crystallized ginger	1/4 cup	60 mL
Hard margarine (or butter), melted	1/4 cup	60 mL
All-purpose flour	2 cups	500 mL
Baking powder	1 tsp.	5 mL
Baking soda	1/4 tsp.	1 mL
Salt	1/4 tsp.	1 mL
Ground cinnamon	1/4 tsp.	1 mL
Ground nutmeg	1/8 tsp.	0.5 mL

Place tea bag in heatproof medium bowl. Pour boiling water over top. Cover. Let steep for 5 minutes. Squeeze and discard tea bag.

Add next 3 ingredients. Stir. Cover. Let stand for 1 to 2 hours until raisins are softened.

Combine next 5 ingredients in large bowl.

Add raisin mixture and remaining 6 ingredients. Stir until just moistened. Spread evenly in greased 9 x 9 inch (22 x 22 cm) pan. Bake in 350°F (175°C) oven for about 45 minutes until wooden pick inserted in centre comes out clean. Cuts into 9 pieces.

1 piece: 422 Calories; 9.2 g Total Fat (4.4 g Mono, 2.6 g Poly, 1.6 g Sat); 24 mg Cholesterol; 83 g Carbohydrate; 3 g Fibre; 6 g Protein; 237 mg Sodium

Banana Date Waffles

It doesn't get much better than this—unless, of course, you add a dollop of whipped topping!

Brown sugar, packed	1/3 cup	75 mL
2% evaporated milk	3 tbsp.	50 mL
Hard margarine (or butter)	2 tbsp.	30 mL
Medium bananas, cut into 1/4 inch (6 mm) slices	3	3
Chopped pitted dates	1/4 cup	60 mL
Frozen waffles	4	4
Pecan pieces, toasted (see Tip, page 47)	1/4 cup	60 mL

Heat and stir first 3 ingredients in large frying pan on medium for about 3 minutes until margarine is melted and sugar is dissolved.

Add banana and dates. Cook for 3 to 5 minutes, stirring gently, until heated through. Reduce heat to low. Cover to keep warm.

Toast waffles. Place 1 waffle on each of 4 plates. Spoon banana mixture onto each.

Sprinkle with pecans. Serves 4.

1 serving: 397 Calories; 14.8 g Total Fat (8.4 g Mono, 3 g Poly, 2.5 g Sat); 10 mg Cholesterol; 66 g Carbohydrate; 3 g Fibre; 5 g Protein; 381 mg Sodium

 While 100% fruit juice is a good alternative to whole fruits, choose juice that contains pulp to ensure you are getting the benefit of fruit fibre.

Mango Yogurt Swirl

An icy-fresh dessert made with creamy yogurt sweetened with honey.

Cans of sliced mango with syrup (14 oz., 398 mL, each), with syrup	2	2
Lime juice	2 tbsp.	30 mL
Low-fat plain yogurt	1 cup	250 mL
Liquid honey	1/2 cup	125 mL

Process mango with syrup and lime juice in blender or food processor until smooth. Spread evenly in ungreased 2 quart (2 L) shallow baking dish.

Combine yogurt and honey in small bowl. Randomly spoon onto mango mixture. Swirl knife through both mixtures to create marble effect. Cover. Freeze overnight until firm. Scoop into 4 bowls. Serves 4.

1 serving: 379 Calories; 1.3 g Total Fat (0.4 g Mono, 0.1 g Poly, 0.7 g Sat); 4 mg Cholesterol; 95 g Carbohydrate; 2 g Fibre; 4 g Protein; 91 mg Sodium

Pear Cranberry Crumble

Sweet, golden crumble topping invites you to discover delicately sauced fruit. Perfect with frozen yogurt.

Peeled pears, sliced	3	3
Bag of fresh (or frozen) cranberries	12 oz.	340 g
Brown sugar, packed	1/2 cup	125 mL
Minute tapioca	3 tbsp.	50 mL
Lemon juice	2 tsp.	10 mL
CRUMBLE TOPPING		
Quick-cooking rolled oats (not instant)	2/3 cup	150 mL
All-bran cereal	2/3 cup	150 mL
Brown sugar, packed	1/3 cup	75 mL
Ground ginger	1/2 tsp.	2 mL
Ground cinnamon	1/4 tsp.	1 mL
Hard margarine (or butter), cut up	1/2 cup	125 mL

Combine first 5 ingredients in medium bowl. Spread evenly in greased 2 quart (2 L) shallow baking dish.

(continued on next page)

Desserts

Crumble Topping: Combine first 5 ingredients in large bowl. Cut in margarine until mixture resembles coarse crumbs. Sprinkle evenly over pear mixture. Bake in 375°F (190°C) oven for 40 to 45 minutes until pear is tender and topping is browned. Let stand for 15 minutes before serving. Serves 6.

1 serving: 397 Calories; 17.2 g Total Fat (10.7 g Mono, 1.9 g Poly, 3.5 g Sat); 0 mg Cholesterol; 63 g Carbohydrate; 8 g Fibre; 3 g Protein; 275 mg Sodium

PLUM CRANBERRY CRUMBLE: Omit pears. Use 1 1/2 lbs. (680 g) fresh prune plums, pitted and sliced.

 *servings per portion*

Baked Stuffed Apples

Tender apples filled with a zesty fruit and nut stuffing. Serve with a scoop of low-fat ice cream or frozen yogurt for a simple, sweet treat.

Coarsely chopped pecans, toasted (see Tip, page 47)	1/2 cup	125 mL
Golden raisins	1/2 cup	125 mL
Brown sugar, packed	1/2 cup	125 mL
Diced mixed peel	1/4 cup	60 mL
Hard margarine (or butter), softened	3 tbsp.	50 mL
Grated orange zest	2 tsp.	10 mL
Ground cinnamon	1/2 tsp.	2 mL
Large unpeeled tart cooking apples (such as Granny Smith), with peel	6	6
Apple juice	1/2 cup	125 mL

Combine first 7 ingredients in medium bowl.

Carefully remove cores from apples with apple corer, leaving apples whole. Carefully cut around hole in each apple with knife to make hole twice as large. Score peel of each apple in several places (to prevent peel from shrinking). Place apples in greased 3 quart (3 L) shallow baking dish. Spoon pecan mixture into centre of each apple, piling excess on top. Cover top of each with small piece of foil.

Pour apple juice into baking dish around apples. Bake, uncovered, in 350°F (175°C) oven for about 1 hour until apples are tender. Makes 6 stuffed apples.

1 stuffed apple: 350 Calories; 13.4 g Total Fat (8.2 g Mono, 2.5 g Poly, 1.9 g Sat); 0 mg Cholesterol; 61 g Carbohydrate; 5 g Fibre; 2 g Protein; 78 mg Sodium

Anise Rum Pears

Golden pears glisten with caramel-coloured syrup. A wonderful blend of flavours to awaken the taste buds! Serve with low-fat ice cream or frozen yogurt.

Medium pears	4	4
Water	2 cups	500 mL
Brown sugar, packed	3/4 cup	175 mL
Spiced rum	1/3 cup	75 mL
Ground ginger	1 tsp.	5 mL
Whole green cardamom, bruised (see Tip, below)	4	4
Star anise	2	2

Carefully remove cores from pears with apple corer, leaving pears whole (see Note). Peel pears.

Combine remaining 6 ingredients in medium saucepan. Cook on medium for about 5 minutes, stirring occasionally, until sugar is dissolved. Carefully lay pears on side in rum mixture. Bring to a boil. Reduce heat to medium-low. Simmer, uncovered, for about 20 minutes, turning pears occasionally with wooden spoon or rubber spatula, until tender. Remove pears with slotted spoon to medium bowl. Cover to keep warm. Bring rum mixture to a boil on high. Boil gently, uncovered, for about 15 minutes until reduced to about 2/3 cup (150 mL). Discard cardamom and star anise. Place 1 pear on each of 4 dessert plates. Drizzle rum mixture over each. Serves 4.

1 serving: 265 Calories; 0.1 g Total Fat (0 g Mono, 0 g Poly, 0 g Sat); 0 mg Cholesterol; 57 g Carbohydrate; 4 g Fibre; 0 g Protein; 21 mg Sodium

Note: Core pears from bottom with apple corer. A grapefruit knife or melon baller also works well. Cut a small slice from bottom of each pear so they will stand upright on plates.

 To bruise cardamom, pound pods with mallet or press with flat side of wide knife to "bruise," or crack them open slightly.

Mixed Berry Sorbet

A vibrant, raspberry-coloured, icy dessert. Refreshing after a full meal. Serve with fresh berries or sliced kiwifruit.

Water	1 1/4 cups	300 mL
Granulated sugar	1/4 cup	60 mL
Frozen mixed berries	2 cups	500 mL
Water	3 tbsp.	50 mL
Orange liqueur	2 tbsp.	30 mL
Lemon juice	2 tsp.	10 mL
Egg whites (large), see Safety Tip	2	2

Heat and stir first amount of water and sugar in small saucepan on medium for about 2 minutes until sugar is dissolved. Bring to a boil on medium-high. Boil gently for 10 minutes. Cool.

Combine berries and second amount of water in medium saucepan. Cook on medium for about 3 minutes, stirring occasionally, until berries are softened and broken up. Press through sieve into medium bowl. Discard seeds. Add berries to sugar mixture.

Add liqueur and lemon juice. Stir well. Spread evenly in ungreased 1 1/2 quart (1.5 L) shallow baking dish. Freeze for about 2 hours until almost firm.

Beat egg whites in separate medium bowl until soft peaks form. Scrape frozen berry mixture into egg whites. Fold until no white streaks remain. Spread evenly in same baking dish. Freeze for about 2 hours until firm. Scrape mixture into blender or food processor. Process until smooth. Spread evenly in same baking dish. Cover. Freeze for about 2 hours until firm. Serves 4.

1 serving: 118 Calories; 0.3 g Total Fat (0 g Mono, 0.1 g Poly, 0 g Sat); 0 mg Cholesterol; 24 g Carbohydrate; 3 g Fibre; 2 g Protein; 28 mg Sodium

Pictured on page 143.

Safety Tip: This recipe contains uncooked eggs. Make sure to use fresh, clean Grade A eggs. Keep frozen until consumed. Pregnant women, young children or the elderly are not advised to eat anything containing raw egg.

Rhubarb "Pie"

Crisp, golden phyllo blankets gently sweet rhubarb sauce. Just sweet enough. Beautiful!

Fresh (or frozen) rhubarb, cut into 1/2 inch (12 mm) pieces	6 cups	1.5 L
Granulated sugar	1 cup	250 mL
Water	1/4 cup	60 mL
Grated orange zest	1 tsp.	5 mL
Ground cinnamon	1/2 tsp.	2 mL
Phyllo pastry sheets, thawed according to package directions	6	6
Icing (confectioner's) sugar	1 tsp.	5 mL

Combine first 5 ingredients in large saucepan. Bring to a boil on medium. Reduce heat to medium-low. Simmer, uncovered, for 12 to 15 minutes, stirring occasionally, until rhubarb starts to break up and sauce is thickened. Spread evenly in ungreased 9 inch (22 cm) deep dish pie plate.

Work with pastry sheets 1 at a time. Keep remaining sheets covered with damp tea towel to prevent drying. Spray 1 side of sheet with cooking spray. Loosely bunch. Place on top of rhubarb mixture near edge of pie plate. Spray second sheet with cooking spray. Loosely bunch. Place on top of rhubarb mixture, touching first sheet. Repeat with remaining sheets until rhubarb mixture is completely covered. Spray top of pastry with cooking spray. Bake in 350°F (175°C) oven for about 20 minutes until pastry is crisp and golden. Let stand for 10 minutes.

Sprinkle with icing sugar. Serve warm. Serves 6.

1 serving: 223 Calories; 1.4 g Total Fat (0.3 g Mono, 0.7 g Poly, 0.2 g Sat); 0 mg Cholesterol; 52 g Carbohydrate; 0 g Fibre; 3 g Protein; 149 mg Sodium

Mango Melon Sorbet

A delightfully tangy dessert for a summer barbecue, or for a day when you just need to chill.

Cubed cantaloupe	2 cups	500 mL
Large mango, cubed	1	1
Granulated sugar	1/4 cup	60 mL
Lime juice	1/4 cup	60 mL

(continued on next page)

138   Desserts

Spread cantaloupe in single layer on plastic wrap-lined baking sheet. Freeze for about 1 1/2 hours until firm. Transfer to blender or food processor.

Add remaining 3 ingredients. Process until smooth. Spread evenly in ungreased 1 1/2 quart (1.5 L) shallow baking dish. Cover with plastic wrap. Freeze for about 2 hours until almost firm. Scrape and stir to break up ice crystals. Freeze until firm. Place in refrigerator for 1 hour before serving (to soften slightly). Serves 6.

1 serving: 90 Calories; 0.3 g Total Fat (0.1 g Mono, 0 g Poly, 0 g Sat); 0 mg Cholesterol; 23 g Carbohydrate; 1 g Fibre; 1 g Protein; 6 mg Sodium

Pictured on page 143.

Lime Bananas

A tropical treat that's oh, so sweet. Yum!

Brown sugar, packed	1/3 cup	75 mL
Lime juice	2 tbsp.	30 mL
Grated lime zest	1 tsp.	5 mL
Small bananas, cut into 1 inch (2.5 cm) slices	4	4
Vanilla frozen yogurt	1 cup	250 mL
Sliced almonds, toasted (see Tip, page 47)	2 tbsp.	30 mL

Combine first 3 ingredients in medium frying pan. Add banana. Stir until coated. Cook on medium for 5 to 6 minutes, stirring gently, until banana is softened and sugar is dissolved.

Scoop 1/4 cup (60 mL) frozen yogurt into each of 4 bowls. Spoon banana mixture onto frozen yogurt.

Sprinkle with almonds. Serves 4.

1 serving: 215 Calories; 3.4 g Total Fat (1.6 g Mono, 0.6 g Poly, 0.9 g Sat); 1 mg Cholesterol; 48 g Carbohydrate; 2 g Fibre; 2 g Protein; 17 mg Sodium

Paré Pointer

Ghosts like their eggs terri-fried.

Fruity Bread Pudding

Spongy pudding loaded with pear and blueberries and spiced with nutmeg. Delicious warm or cold.

Chopped, peeled fresh pear	2 cups	500 mL
Fresh (or frozen, thawed) blueberries	1 cup	250 mL
Day-old bread slices, cut into 1/2 inch (12 mm) cubes	8	8
Large eggs	4	4
Milk	2 cups	500 mL
Granulated sugar	1/2 cup	125 mL
Vanilla	1 tsp.	5 mL
Ground nutmeg	1/2 tsp.	2 mL
Coarse brown sugar	2 tbsp.	30 mL

Scatter 1 cup (250 mL) pear and 1/2 cup (125 mL) blueberries in greased 2 quart (2 L) shallow baking dish.

Scatter bread cubes evenly over fruit. Scatter remaining pear and blueberries evenly over bread cubes.

Beat next 5 ingredients with whisk in medium bowl. Carefully pour over top. Let stand for 10 minutes.

Sprinkle with brown sugar. Place baking dish in 9 x 13 inch (22 x 33 cm) pan. Pour boiling water into pan until halfway up side of baking dish. Bake, uncovered, in 325°F (160°C) oven for about 1 1/4 hours until just set. Carefully remove baking dish from pan. Let stand for 20 minutes before serving. Serves 6.

1 serving: 297 Calories; 5.6 g Total Fat (2.1 g Mono, 0.7 g Poly, 1.9 g Sat); 147 mg Cholesterol; 52 g Carbohydrate; 3 g Fibre; 10 g Protein; 269 mg Sodium

 Many fruits are good sources of fibre and vitamins A and C. Make sure to eat the skin (when possible) for the optimum nutritional boost.

Desserts

Apple Carrot Cake

A delicious, moist cake made with applesauce instead of cooking oil. A twist on tradition, but just as good.

All-purpose flour	1 1/2 cups	375 mL
Whole-wheat flour	1/2 cup	125 mL
Baking soda	2 tsp.	10 mL
Ground cinnamon	1 1/2 tsp.	7 mL
Ground nutmeg	1/2 tsp.	2 mL
Salt	1 tsp.	5 mL
Large eggs	4	4
Grated carrot	2 cups	500 mL
Grated peeled cooking apple (such as McIntosh)	1 1/2 cups	375 mL
Applesauce	1 cup	250 mL
Granulated sugar	1 cup	250 mL
Golden raisins	1 cup	250 mL
APPLE CREAM ICING		
Icing (confectioner's) sugar	1 cup	250 mL
Light cream cheese, softened	4 oz.	125 g
Hard margarine (or butter), softened	1/4 cup	60 mL
Frozen concentrated apple juice	2 tbsp.	30 mL

Measure first 6 ingredients into large bowl. Stir. Make a well in centre.

Combine next 6 ingredients in separate large bowl. Add to well. Stir until just moistened. Spread evenly in greased 9 x 13 inch (22 x 33 cm) pan. Bake in 350°F (175°C) oven for about 45 minutes until wooden pick inserted in centre comes out clean. Let stand in pan on wire rack to cool completely.

Apple Cream Icing: Beat all 4 ingredients in medium bowl on medium until smooth. Makes about 1 1/2 cups (375 mL) icing. Spread evenly on top of cake in pan. Cuts into 12 pieces.

1 piece: 342 Calories; 8.2 g Total Fat (3.9 g Mono, 0.9 g Poly, 2.6 g Sat); 78 mg Cholesterol; 63 g Carbohydrate; 3 g Fibre; 6 g Protein; 563 mg Sodium

Pictured on page 36.

Peachsicle Slice

Golden layers of peachy frozen yogurt sandwich vanilla ice cream. Serve with fresh berries or berry coulis (COO-lee), or fruit purée.

Orange juice	2 cups	500 mL
Chopped dried peaches	1/2 cup	125 mL
Can of sliced peaches in pear juice (with juice)	14 oz.	398 mL
Low-fat peach yogurt	1/2 cup	125 mL
Low-fat vanilla ice cream, softened	1 1/2 cups	375 mL

Process orange juice and dried peaches in blender or food processor until smooth.

Add canned peaches and yogurt. Process until smooth. Spread half of mixture evenly in plastic wrap-lined 9 x 5 x 3 inch (22 x 12.5 x 7.5 cm) loaf pan. Freeze for about 3 hours until firm. Chill remaining peach mixture.

Spread ice cream evenly on top of frozen peach mixture. Stir chilled peach mixture. Spread evenly on top of ice cream. Cover. Freeze overnight until firm. Invert onto cutting board. Discard plastic wrap. Cuts into 8 slices (see Note).

1 slice: 173 Calories; 3.2 g Total Fat (0.9 g Mono, 0.2 g Poly, 1.8 g Sat); 12 mg Cholesterol; 36 g Carbohydrate; 3 g Fibre; 3 g Protein; 37 mg Sodium

Pictured at right.

Note: To easily cut frozen desserts, dip knife in hot water before cutting each slice.

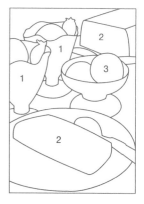

1. Mixed Berry Sorbet, page 137
2. Peachsicle Slice, above
3. Mango Melon Sorbet, page 138

Props courtesy of: Canhome Global
Casa Bugatti

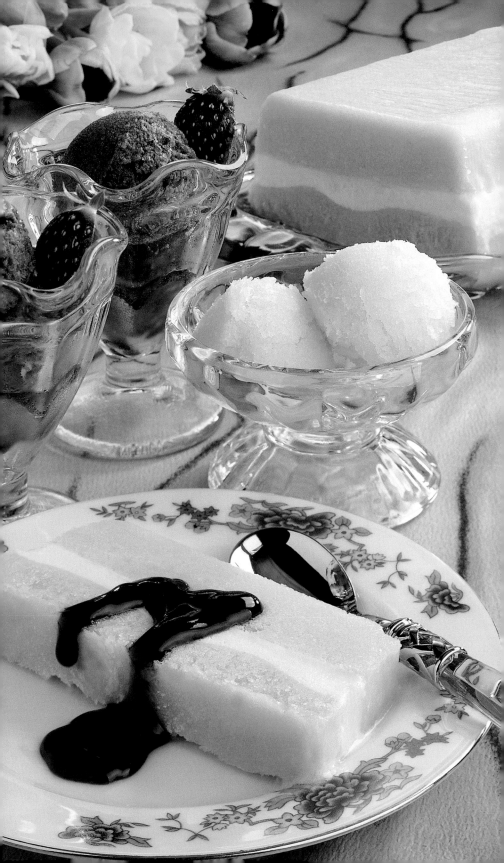

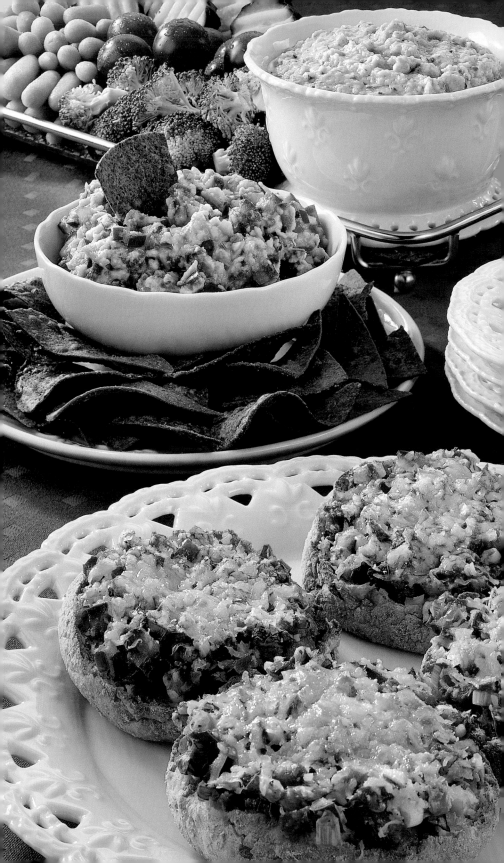

Spiced Eggplant Dip

Chunky dip with flecks of herbs and a subtle chili flavour. Something a little different to serve with tortilla chips.

Eggplant	1	1
Coarse dry bread crumbs	1/2 cup	125 mL
Water	1/4 cup	60 mL
Low-fat plain yogurt	1/3 cup	75 mL
Chopped fresh parsley	2 tbsp.	30 mL
(or 1 1/2 tsp., 7 mL, flakes)		
Lemon juice	1 tbsp.	15 mL
Sweet chili sauce	1 tbsp.	15 mL
Ground cumin	1/2 tsp.	2 mL
Chili powder	1/4 tsp.	1 mL

Randomly poke several holes with fork into eggplant. Place on greased baking sheet. Bake in 350°F (175°C) oven for about 40 minutes until softened. Remove from oven. Let stand on baking sheet for about 10 minutes until cool enough to handle. Cut eggplant in half. Scrape flesh into blender or food processor. Discard peel.

Combine bread crumbs and water in small bowl. Let stand for about 5 minutes until water is absorbed. Add to eggplant.

Add remaining 6 ingredients. Process until smooth. Serves 4.

1 serving: 100 Calories; 1.4 g Total Fat (0.4 g Mono, 0.3 g Poly, 0.4 g Sat); 1 mg Cholesterol; 19 g Carbohydrate; 3 g Fibre; 4 g Protein; 140 mg Sodium

Pictured at left.

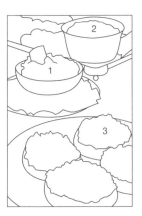

1. Special Guacamole, page 146
2. Spiced Eggplant Dip, above
3. English Bruschetta, page 147

Props courtesy of: Cherison Enterprises Inc.

Date Apple Cheese Snack

A sweet, crunchy combination. Add more honey if you like your snacks a little sweeter.
Serve on a bed of lettuce.

Peeled large cooking apple (such as McIntosh), chopped	1	1
1% cottage cheese	1/2 cup	125 mL
Chopped pitted dates	1/4 cup	60 mL
Pecan pieces, toasted (see Tip, page 47)	2 tbsp.	30 mL
Raw sunflower seeds, toasted (see Tip, page 47)	2 tbsp.	30 mL
Liquid honey	1 tbsp.	15 mL

Combine all 6 ingredients in small bowl. Serves 2.

1 serving: 299 Calories; 10.9 g Total Fat (4.3 g Mono, 4.5 g Poly, 1.4 g Sat); 3 mg Cholesterol; 45 g Carbohydrate; 4 g Fibre; 10 g Protein; 251 mg Sodium

Special Guacamole

Creamy avocado and juicy tomatoes make a delightful dip. Colourful and zesty—perfect for taco chips.

Ripe large avocado	1	1
Finely chopped green onion	1 tbsp.	15 mL
Lime juice	1 tbsp.	15 mL
Finely chopped jalapeño pepper (see Tip, page 117)	2 tsp.	10 mL
Garlic clove, minced (or 1/4 tsp., 1 mL, powder)	1	1
Ground cumin	1/4 tsp.	1 mL
Pepper, sprinkle		
Medium tomatoes, seeds removed, finely chopped	2	2

Mash avocado in medium bowl. Add next 6 ingredients. Mix well.

Add tomato. Stir. Serves 6.

1 serving: 76 Calories; 6.3 g Total Fat (3.9 g Mono, 0.8 g Poly, 1 g Sat); 0 mg Cholesterol; 5 g Carbohydrate; 2 g Fibre; 1 g Protein; 8 mg Sodium

Pictured on page 144.

English Bruschetta

Tasty bruschetta made with toasted English muffins and seasoned with a little cumin to make them interesting. "Cumin" get 'em!

Medium tomatoes, seeds removed, finely chopped	2	2
Finely chopped green onion	2 tbsp.	30 mL
Chopped fresh basil (or 1 1/2 tsp., 7 mL, dried)	2 tbsp.	30 mL
Red wine vinegar	1 tsp.	5 mL
Ground cumin	1/8 tsp.	0.5 mL
Pepper	1/8 tsp.	0.5 mL
Whole-wheat English muffins, split	2	2
Grated Parmesan cheese	1/4 cup	60 mL

Combine first 6 ingredients in small bowl.

Toast both halves of each muffin. Place muffins, split-side up, on ungreased baking sheet. Spoon tomato mixture onto each half.

Sprinkle Parmesan cheese over each. Broil 6 inches (15 cm) from heat for 2 to 3 minutes until Parmesan cheese is melted and starts to brown. Makes 4 bruschetta. Serves 2.

1 serving: 218 Calories; 5.6 g Total Fat (1.4 g Mono, 0.8 g Poly, 2.8 g Sat); 10 mg Cholesterol; 33 g Carbohydrate; 2 g Fibre; 12 g Protein; 478 mg Sodium

Pictured on page 144.

Paré Pointer

Insects travel in an old-fashioned way—they prefer buggy rides.

Fruit-Full Muffins

*Moist, tender muffins full of tangy rhubarb and cranberries, topped with sweet crumbs.
Just as good without the topping.*

Large egg, fork-beaten	1	1
Chopped fresh (or frozen, thawed) rhubarb	1 1/2 cups	375 mL
Chopped fresh (or frozen, thawed) strawberries	1 1/2 cups	375 mL
Dried cranberries	1 cup	250 mL
Unsweetened applesauce	1 cup	250 mL
Hard margarine (or butter), melted	1/2 cup	125 mL
All-purpose flour	3 cups	750 mL
Brown sugar, packed	1 cup	250 mL
Baking soda	1 tsp.	5 mL
Salt	1/2 tsp.	2 mL
NUTTY TOPPING		
Brown sugar, packed	1/4 cup	60 mL
Ground walnuts	1 tbsp.	15 mL
Ground cinnamon	1/4 tsp.	1 mL

Combine first 6 ingredients in large bowl.

Combine next 4 ingredients in separate large bowl. Make a well in centre. Add fruit mixture to well. Stir until just moistened. Grease 12 muffin cups with cooking spray. Fill cups full.

Nutty Topping: Combine all 3 ingredients in small bowl. Sprinkle evenly over muffins. Bake in 375°F (190°C) oven for 20 to 25 minutes until wooden pick inserted in centre of muffin comes out clean. Let stand in pan for 5 minutes before removing to wire rack to cool. Makes 12 muffins.

1 muffin: 324 Calories; 8.8 g Total Fat (5.3 g Mono, 1.1 g Poly, 1.7 g Sat); 0 mg Cholesterol; 59 g Carbohydrate; 3 g Fibre; 4 g Protein; 312 mg Sodium

Pictured on page 125 and on back cover.

Antipasto

Colourful and chunky. Serve with crisped baguette slices or your favourite crackers. Freezes well.

Cooking oil	2 tbsp.	30 mL
Chopped cauliflower florets	1 cup	250 mL
Finely chopped onion	1/4 cup	60 mL
Small garlic clove, minced	1	1
Diced green pepper	1/2 cup	125 mL
Diced red pepper	1/2 cup	125 mL
Can of mushroom stems and pieces, drained and chopped	10 oz.	284 mL
Ketchup	1 cup	250 mL
Can of sliced black olives, drained	4 1/2 oz.	125 mL
Chopped gherkin (or dill pickle)	1/4 cup	60 mL
Gherkin (or dill pickle) juice	2 tbsp.	30 mL
Can of flaked tuna, drained	6 oz.	170 g

Heat cooking oil in large saucepan on medium. Add next 3 ingredients. Cook for 5 to 10 minutes, stirring often, until onion is softened.

Add green and red pepper. Cook for about 5 minutes, stirring occasionally, until pepper is softened.

Add next 5 ingredients. Stir. Mixture will be very thick. Bring to a boil. Boil gently, uncovered, for 5 minutes, stirring often. Reduce heat to medium-low. Heat and stir for 5 minutes.

Add tuna. Stir well. Remove from heat. Cool. Chill for at least 3 hours until cold. Makes about 3 cups (750 mL). Serves 6.

1 serving: 148 Calories; 5.9 g Total Fat (3.4 g Mono, 1.7 g Poly, 0.5 g Sat); 8 mg Cholesterol; 18 g Carbohydrate; 2 g Fibre; 8 g Protein; 895 mg Sodium

Measurement Tables

Throughout this book measurements are given in Conventional and Metric measure. To compensate for differences between the two measurements due to rounding, a full metric measure is not always used. The cup used is the standard 8 fluid ounce. Temperature is given in degrees Fahrenheit and Celsius. Baking pan measurements are in inches and centimetres as well as quarts and litres. An exact metric conversion is given below as well as the working equivalent (Metric Standard Measure).

Spoons

Conventional Measure	Metric Exact Conversion Millilitre (mL)	Metric Standard Measure Millilitre (mL)
1/8 teaspoon (tsp.)	0.6 mL	0.5 mL
1/4 teaspoon (tsp.)	1.2 mL	1 mL
1/2 teaspoon (tsp.)	2.4 mL	2 mL
1 teaspoon (tsp.)	4.7 mL	5 mL
2 teaspoons (tsp.)	9.4 mL	10 mL
1 tablespoon (tbsp.)	14.2 mL	15 mL

Cups

Conventional Measure	Metric Exact Conversion Millilitre (mL)	Metric Standard Measure Millilitre (mL)
1/4 cup (4 tbsp.)	56.8 mL	60 mL
1/3 cup (5 1/3 tbsp.)	75.6 mL	75 mL
1/2 cup (8 tbsp.)	113.7 mL	125 mL
2/3 cup (10 2/3 tbsp.)	151.2 mL	150 mL
3/4 cup (12 tbsp.)	170.5 mL	175 mL
1 cup (16 tbsp.)	227.3 mL	250 mL
4 1/2 cups	1022.9 mL	1000 mL (1 L)

Oven Temperatures

Fahrenheit (°F)	Celsius (°C)
175°	80°
200°	95°
225°	110°
250°	120°
275°	140°
300°	150°
325°	160°
350°	175°
375°	190°
400°	205°
425°	220°
450°	230°
475°	240°
500°	260°

Dry Measurements

Conventional Measure Ounces (oz.)	Metric Exact Conversion Grams (g)	Metric Standard Measure Grams (g)
1 oz.	28.3 g	28 g
2 oz.	56.7 g	57 g
3 oz.	85.0 g	85 g
4 oz.	113.4 g	125 g
5 oz.	141.7 g	140 g
6 oz.	170.1 g	170 g
7 oz.	198.4 g	200 g
8 oz.	226.8 g	250 g
16 oz.	453.6 g	500 g
32 oz.	907.2 g	1000 g (1 kg)

Pans

Conventional Inches	Metric Centimetres
8x8 inch	20x20 cm
9x9 inch	22x22 cm
9x13 inch	22x33 cm
10x15 inch	25x38 cm
11x17 inch	28x43 cm
8x2 inch round	20x5 cm
9x2 inch round	22x5 cm
10x4 1/2 inch tube	25x11 cm
8x4x3 inch loaf	20x10x7.5 cm
9x5x3 inch loaf	22x12.5x7.5 cm

Casseroles

CANADA & BRITAIN		UNITED STATES	
Standard Size Casserole	Exact Metric Measure	Standard Size Casserole	Exact Metric Measure
1 qt. (5 cups)	1.13 L	1 qt. (4 cups)	900 mL
1 1/2 qts. (7 1/2 cups)	1.69 L	1 1/2 qts. (6 cups)	1.35 L
2 qts. (10 cups)	2.25 L	2 qts. (8 cups)	1.8 L
2 1/2 qts. (12 1/2 cups)	2.81 L	2 1/2 qts. (10 cups)	2.25 L
3 qts. (15 cups)	3.38 L	3 qts. (12 cups)	2.7 L
4 qts. (20 cups)	4.5 L	4 qts. (16 cups)	3.6 L
5 qts. (25 cups)	5.63 L	5 qts. (20 cups)	4.5 L

Recipe Index

152

153

Q

R

S

154

155

156

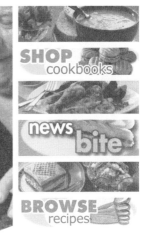

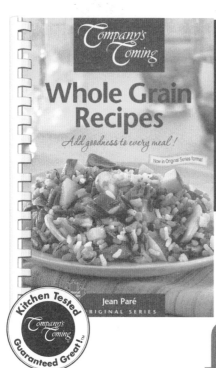

Try it

a sample recipe from *Whole Grain Recipes*

Buckwheat Sunrise

Whole Grain Recipes, Page 37

Water	1 1/2 cups	375 mL
Whole buckwheat	1 cup	250 mL
Grated orange zest	1 tsp.	5 mL
Salt	1/4 tsp.	1 mL
Orange juice	1 cup	250 mL
Chopped dried apricot	1/3 cup	75 mL
Dried cranberries	1/3 cup	75 mL
Liquid honey	3 tbsp.	50 mL
Slivered almonds, toasted	1/4 cup	60 mL

1 cup (250 mL): 367 Calories; 6.1 g Total Fat (3.3 g Mono, 1.6 g Poly, 0.7 g Sat); 0 mg Cholesterol; 76 g Carbohydrate; 6 g Fibre; 8 g Protein; 210 mg Sodium

Variation: Instead of dried cranberries, use same amount of chopped dried cherries.

Combine first 4 ingredients in medium saucepan. Bring to a boil. Reduce heat to medium-low. Simmer, covered, for about 15 minutes, without stirring, until buckwheat is tender.

Add orange juice. Stir. Add next 3 ingredients. Stir. Transfer to medium bowl. Cool at room temperature before covering. Chill for at least 6 hours or overnight until apricot and cranberries are softened and liquid is absorbed.

Add almonds. Stir. Makes about 3 cups (750 mL).

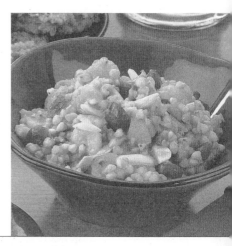

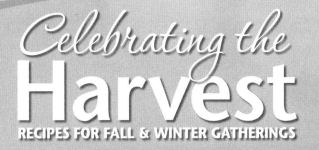

Celebrating the
Harvest
RECIPES FOR FALL & WINTER GATHERINGS

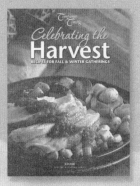

Whether from the garden, farmers' market or supermarket, harvest ingredients display the bounty and beauty of nature. Entertain a crowd in style, or feed your family comfort food they'll not soon forget—with new delicious recipes that celebrate harvest ingredients. What a lovely way to get through the long fall and winter!

SPECIAL OCCASION SERIES

If you like what we've done with **cooking**, you'll **love** what we do with **crafts!**

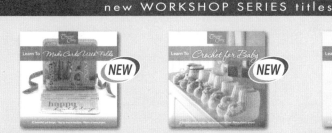

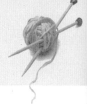